Praise for Juan Carlos Santana

"Juan Carlos 'JC' Santana is the preeminent personal trainer, period! *Functional Training* will provide you with key insights into the science and application of exercise training."

Jose Antonio, PhD, CEO of ISSN

"Juan Carlos 'JC' Santana is the premier trainer in America, and *Functional Training* is groundbreaking work in the area of function and strength. There is simply no better resource on the planet."

Lee E. Brown, EdD, CSCS*D, FNSCA, FACSM
Professor, Strength and Conditioning
Director, Center for Sport Performance
California State University, Fullerton
Editor, *Training for Speed, Agility, & Quickness*

"For over 30 years Juan Carlos 'JC' Santana has been raising the bar in the fitness industry. With *Functional Training* you will tap into the cutting-edge methods that have made him one of the world's leading authorities on functional training."

Jeff Chandler, EdD, CSCS*D, NSCA-CPT*D, FNSCA, FACSM
Professor, Jacksonville State University
Editor in Chief, *Strength and Conditioning Journal*

"If you want to reach your potential as an athlete there is no one I would trust more than Juan Carlos 'JC' Santana!"

Mike Flynn
11-Year NFL Veteran
Super Bowl XXXV Champion

"Juan Carlos 'JC' Santana is a fitness leader with a unique understanding of the science and practice of functional training. He creates superior results for duffers and high-performance athletes alike, and his book *Functional Training* will show you how to make the most of your training."

Stuart McGill, PhD
Professor, University of Waterloo at Waterloo, Ontario, Canada

"With Juan Carlos 'JC' Santana's training methods and guidance, I was able to fight at the highest level of mixed martial arts in the UFC and Pride Fighting Championships and reached the pinnacle of grappling by winning the ADCC Submission Wrestling World Championship. The workout regimens in *Functional Training* will also prepare you for any competition."

Jeff "Snowman" Monson
Pro MMA Fighter
ADCC Submission Wrestling World Champion

Functional Training

Juan Carlos Santana

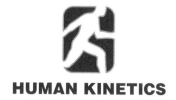

HUMAN KINETICS

Library of Congress Cataloging-in-Publication Data

Santana, Juan Carlos, 1959-
 Functional training / Juan Carlos Santana.
    pages cm
 Includes index.
 1. Physical education and training. 2. Coaching (Athletics) 3. Athletes--Training of. 4. Exercise.
 I. Title.
 GV711.5.S27 2016
 613.7--dc23
                                         2015015211
 ISBN: 978-1-4504-1482-1 (print)

Acquisitions Editor: Michelle Maloney; **Developmental Editor:** Cynthia McEntire; **Managing Editor:** Elizabeth Evans; **Copyeditor and Indexer:** Alisha Jeddeloh; **Permissions Manager:** Martha Gullo; **Senior Graphic Designer:** Nancy Rasmus; **Cover Designer:** Keith Blomberg; **Photograph (cover):** Rio Santana; **Photographs (interior):** Neil Bernstein; **Photographer's Assistant:** Rio Santana; **Visual Production Assistant:** Joyce Brumfield; **Photo Production Manager:** Jason Allen; **Art Manager:** Kelly Hendren; **Associate Art Manager:** Alan L. Wilborn; **Illustrations:** © Human Kinetics, unless otherwise noted; **Printer:** Sheridan Books

We thank the Institute of Human Performance in Boca Raton, Florida, for assistance in providing the location for the photo shoot for this book.

Human Kinetics books are available at special discounts for bulk purchase. Special editions or book excerpts can also be created to specification. For details, contact the Special Sales Manager at Human Kinetics.

Printed in the United States of America   10 9 8 7 6 5 4 3 2 1

The paper in this book is certified under a sustainable forestry program.

Human Kinetics
Website: www.HumanKinetics.com

United States: Human Kinetics
P.O. Box 5076
Champaign, IL 61825-5076
800-747-4457
e-mail: humank@hkusa.com

Canada: Human Kinetics
475 Devonshire Road Unit 100
Windsor, ON N8Y 2L5
800-465-7301 (in Canada only)
e-mail: info@hkcanada.com

Europe: Human Kinetics
107 Bradford Road
Stanningley
Leeds LS28 6AT, United Kingdom
+44 (0) 113 255 5665
e-mail: hk@hkeurope.com

Australia: Human Kinetics
57A Price Avenue
Lower Mitcham, South Australia 5062
08 8372 0999
e-mail: info@hkaustralia.com

New Zealand: Human Kinetics
P.O. Box 80
Mitcham Shopping Centre, South Australia 5062
0800 222 062
e-mail: info@hknewzealand.com

E5531

This book is dedicated to my children, Rio, Caila, Dante, and Mia, for teaching me the wonders of divine inspiration and unconditional love.

Contents

Acknowledgments

Most of what is learned in college and reinforced by certifications is theoretical information that is better suited for college professors instead of personal trainers, coaches, practicing therapists, or athletes. Schools teach opposite to how humans learn. In life, we learn to practice first; then, if needed, we learn the details. In school, we learn the details first and then work our way to the big concepts. However, in many instances school never quite gets to the practice. We only learn how to practice the skill we went to school to learn once we get out of school and hit the field or training floor.

I have had the great pleasure and honor of sharing the stage with some of the brightest minds in the fitness industry. I have learned much from these industry pioneers, but one thing stands out—if you can't use it on the field or training floor, then it's not much use to a training system. *Functional Training* shares the practical approaches I have used for more than 40 years of my life as an athlete and coach. Although some of the theories and concepts may be complex, I stay away from complicated language and theory when communicating them. Albert Einstein reportedly said, "If you can't explain it simply, you don't know it well enough." This book is my attempt at finding out how well I know my material.

They say it takes a village to raise a child; no truer words have been spoken. I would like to mention some of the key people in my village throughout my life. Many more wonderful people can't be mentioned because of space and time constraints; however, their absence here does not take away from their important influence in my life.

This book is dedicated to my family of origin, who came from Cuba in search of the American dream in 1966: my parents, Celerina and Arnaldo Santana, and my sister, Belkis Olson-Handras. They provided me with nothing but love, understanding, compassion, and guidance; together we found and built the American dream. As children often do, my four children—Rio, Caila, Dante, and Mia—came at key moments in my life, and all have inspired me to be the best man I can be. I have dedicated my life to them and I hope this book serves as a symbol and reminder to them of what is possible with hard work. Children need lots of love from their parents, and I would be remiss in not thanking Annie Aponte for her wonderful role in Rio's upbringing and Debbie Santana for her caring love and attention to the lives of Caila, Dante, and Mia. To my extended family (i.e., Moni, Eric, Lee, and all of my cousins, aunts, and uncles), thank you for being there and making all holidays memorable family reunions. I love you all.

My coaches and teachers—Anthony Abbott, Julia George, Sue Graves, Andy Siegel, and Michael Whitehurst, to name a few—have been instrumental in my continual development, and I can only hope I have a similar impact on my students and athletes. Many thanks to my dear friends Mark Bagg, Pierro Busani, Steve Cannavale, Rocky DePhilipo, Guy Fitzpatrick, Scott Goodpaster, Jeff Harpster, Mark Meade, Roly Ortega, Barry Pavel, Scott Smith, Kado Tundisi, and Dave Woynarowski, to name but a few, for being references, beacons, and points of lights even on my darkest days. I would also like to pay my respects to some people I consider to be giants in the fitness, strength, conditioning, and medical world—Anthony Abbott, Joey Antonio, Tudor Bompa, Lee Brown, Gary Gray, Doug Kalman, William Kraemer, and Stu McGill, to name a few within a very large group. I'm proud to call these individuals friends and colleagues.

Because this book is about functional training, I would be negligent if I did not give a special acknowledgment to Gary Gray, the eminent leader of our modern functional training revolution. Gary's teachings helped mold me into the professional I am today, and his teachings and wisdom are interlaced throughout the pages in this book. No book on functional training can be complete without acknowledging the vision of Chris Poirier and Perform Better. It was Chris's idea to educate the fitness world on functional training, and under his directive Perform Better he launched the longest running functional training education tour in fitness history. It was an honor for me to start that tour with Chris and Perform Better in 1997 and still associate with them today.

My deepest gratitude goes to my Institute of Human Performance (IHP) family for their love and support of what was once only a dream. To them I say, "We did it. We created the best training facility on the planet. What we have created is bigger than any one person and is truly amazing!" The IHP family is made up of *all* members and staff who have passed through our doors and blessed us with their gifts and support. As of the writing of this book, our primary staff is composed of Rio, Lily, Pieri, Grif, Adam, Gabe, Scott, Marc, Pedro, Tamara, Jenna, Georgia, and all of the wonderful interns who make IHP their training headquarters. A big thank-you to all of our IHP models: Tamara Estevez, Pedro Penaherrera, Gabriel Saavedra, Marc Saint-Preux, Rio Santana, Jared Stan, and Jenna Worswick. IHP's international representatives must also be acknowledged for their faith in IHP and their willingness to take our message beyond our borders. These international reps—Justo and Marisa Aon, Connie Beaulieu, Fernando Jaeger, Luis Noya, Ruben Payan, Eduardo and Kimberly Poveda, and Joel Proskowitz —have been instrumental in launching the IHP global family. Together we have made IHP a worldwide brand. Thank you.

Finally, I want to thank a very special person in my life, Jessica "Chuli" Lozano, for her role in my personal and spiritual evolution.

Introduction

Over the last two decades, training and conditioning methods have evolved at a mind-blistering pace. World records have fallen, rehabilitation times have been practically cut in half, and athletes in their 40s are now competing in professional sports once thought the domain of younger athletes. Even weekend athletes are competing at levels once considered professional. What has made this rapid improvement possible? Nutrition and skill training have certainly played a huge role in the dramatic improvements we see on the playing field. However, the biggest changes have occurred in training. If you look at diet, supplements, and skill training, the basics are still the same. However, when it comes to training, the amount of new information is coming so fast that research and traditional education can't keep pace with it. Never in our history have we had more choices of exercises, equipment, and training approaches.

One of the most popular training philosophies to evolve over the last 25 years is functional training. Although a single definition is yet to be universally accepted, functional training develops functional strength specific to a given activity. Until recently, professional trainers and coaches were the only people who had access to educational resources that explained the methods of functional training. Fitness conferences and seminars, DVDs, and books were the only ways you could learn about functional training from an experienced practitioner. However, over the last 15 years the philosophy of functional training has evolved into something quite different. If you pick up any popular magazine, you will find a slew of functional training exercises and programs. Spend one hour on YouTube or Facebook and you can watch hundreds of exercises performed in the name of functional training. The only problem with all of this information in the popular press and online is that many of the so-called experts writing these articles and posting videos have short résumés in the field and in exercise science as it pertains to functional training. In some instances, the only qualifications are active Facebook and Twitter pages and thousands of hits on YouTube.

The modern evolution of functional training is fascinating. In my lifetime, I have witnessed the physical preparation process go through a metamorphosis that rivals the *Rocky* sequels. We have gone from purely functional and sport-specific training to high-priced training gadgets. At the same time, our culture has gone from preferring a slim athletic look to celebrating muscle-packed speed demons. These two separate worlds of performance and culture continue to interact and influence how books, such as this one, are written.

Once upon a time everything was functional and all training was functional. If you were an athlete in a sport that did not require lots of strength but did require lots of skill (e.g., tennis, golf, swimming), you practiced your sport until you were better than everyone else. Even if you practiced a sport that required lots of strength (e.g., track and field thrower, American football lineman, heavyweight boxer), you simply did some strength training in the off-season or chopped lots of logs with a heavy ax in preparation for a fight.

When I was a young man in the late 1960s and early 1970s, there were no high-tech machines. We worshipped the great athletes such as Babe Ruth and Joe Lewis. We were taught that these low-tech, high-touch performers were born athletic, and hard skill work forged the player. The strength training and conditioning of these athletes was minimal by most standards and very skill oriented. For example, Babe Ruth was not known for doing much training, but his accomplishments are etched in stone. Joe Lewis did not do anything out of the ordinary to prepare for fights, but his warrior spirit carried him into the history books.

Much of what I grew up doing as a young martial artist was what we would today call *functional training*. The popular fitness personalities of my era, such as Jack LaLanne and Bruce Lee, advocated a functional approach to training that involved mostly calisthenics and standard cardio (running on various surfaces and skipping rope). Jack LaLanne prepared for his famous swims by tugging boats while swimming. Bruce Lee prepared for his famous 1-inch (3 cm) punch by doing one-arm, two-finger push-ups.

As times changed and so did technology, functional training took a back seat to the more popular bodybuilding methods of the 1980s. The era of Arnold Schwarzenegger and pumping iron gave birth to new methods of physical preparation. Training during this time mostly consisted of traditional strength training, with functional training taking a backseat. Although functional training systems never quite died, they were difficult to find. The bodybuilding approach was used to prepare for sports, and weight rooms across the world stocked up on iron. During this era every athlete from every sport got bigger. The no-name defense of the 1972 Miami Dolphins gave way to the Steel Curtain of the Pittsburgh Steelers, the Rocky Marciano build gave way to the stature of George Foreman and Evander Holyfield, and Jesse Owens was transformed into Ben Johnson.

The clash between the skilled speed needed for better performance and the bigger physiques created by bodybuilding-dominated training was problematic for many sports. Injuries begin to plague the sports arena, and many athletes felt their performances were compromised by the additional muscle that bodybuilding produced. Some skill-dominated sports begin to shy away from weightlifting, and the demand for alternative training methods that could rehabilitate injuries and improve performance without building muscle brought functional training back to center stage. The 1990s and early years of the new millennium saw an explosion in functional training. For instance, Evander Holyfield put on almost 40 pounds (18 kg) of solid muscle by training with Lee Haney and Dr. Hatfield. This massive increase in size was accompanied by an increase in speed, agility, and quickness thanks to the functional training provided by Tim Hallmark.

Even within the small circle of functional training pioneers, many theories and practices have changed. What we thought were effective functional training methods 20 years ago now are rarely used, and what we thought were outdated and ineffective training methods now take center stage. We have witnessed this evolution firsthand in our training facility, the Institute of Human Performance (IHP). Over the last 14 years, we have seen equipment lines come and go, we have seen toys and gadgets come and go, and we have seen panacea methods come and go. If I had to sum up the last 15 years, I would say this: We are back to basics!

Today, it is hard to find an athlete or strength and conditioning coach who doesn't claim to use functional training. Although the term *functional training* had already been used by therapy and fitness pioneers for many decades, it was first popularized by the media in the 1990s and its popularity has grown ever since. I still remember my first interview with *Men's Journal* on the topic of functional training. They asked me for a functional exercise and I showed them the single-leg anterior reach Gary Gray had shown me a few months before. That issue was published in 1998, and since then just about every major magazine has contacted me to provide them with functional training exercises and protocols. Welcome to the commercialization of functional training!

The commercialization of functional training has been matched and raised, as they say in poker. Due to the Internet and infomercials, what was originally a revolution based on legitimate practice has become an atomic blast of confusion and self-proclaimed expertise. Facebook, YouTube, and Twitter have created Internet experts, e-book authors, and iMovie video producers. You can go to YouTube and watch hours of something called *functional training*, but you will see nothing short of exercises that can qualify as entertaining circus acts, mostly ineffective and often dangerous. Even national conferences that once extensively vetted all presenters now take people who have a huge Facebook following but little experience or formal education. Enter the era of confusion, where everyone is an expert, everything is functional, and nobody knows where the myths got started.

This book is an attempt to provide some clarity where there seems to be little. We provide scientific references when necessary, but most importantly we provide a logical approach to function and functional training. We don't want you to believe what we are proposing; we want you to know it is so because it makes so much sense!

Functional Training brings you up-to-date definitions of functional training, breakthroughs in the field, specific exercises, and sport-specific training programs. Its concepts and training methods are safe, effective, and scientifically sound. Although the concepts are sophisticated, they are presented in a straightforward manner that any trainer, coach, therapist, athlete, or parent will understand. The book is simple enough to be understood by high school athletes and their parents but sophisticated and effective enough to be of interest to personal trainers and strength coaches.

The organization of *Functional Training* follows a logical path to provide a basic but comprehensive understanding of this popular topic. The book is divided into three parts. Part I provides a historical background of strength training, along with definitions of the key elements of function and functional training. Chapter 1 begins with a brief history of the fitness industry and functional training. Then it provides operational definitions of *function* and *functional training* so we all are on the same page. The discussion proceeds to the logical, scientific reasons why functional training is so effective, and it provides some best-practice applications. The chapter concludes by reviewing popular equipment used in commercial gyms, home studios, and parks and while traveling.

Chapter 2 covers the basic movement skills in most sports and explains how the body is designed for those skills. The discussion then turns to the training octagon and how to base an athletic functional training system on this training model. Next comes a discussion of the operational environment of sport and how the physical qualities of that environment affect movement and functional training. The chapter concludes by explaining how the body uses neural input from the physical world and its own movement to create efficient and coordinated movement sequences.

Chapter 3 introduces the performance continuum, a simple strategy to guide you through the process of beginning functional training and progressing based on successful, controlled movements. This chapter also outlines some simple techniques for manipulating the intensity of functional exercises so that they match the athlete's ability.

Part II covers functional modalities and the most useful functional exercises within each modality. Chapter 4 includes exercises that use body weight, bands and cables, and dumbbells and kettlebells. Chapter 5 adds exercises that use medicine balls, stability balls, and new training toys, and it even includes traditional strength exercises. It outlines the advantages of each modality and gives instructions for the most popular exercises.

Part III discusses the fundamentals of exercise selection, programming, and periodization and provides sample programs for common sports. Chapter 6 discusses the fundamental elements of program design and periodization as they relate to functional training and strength development. Functional training programs for all four major periodization cycles are presented in template form to facilitate easy substitution of exercises. Chapter 7 provides strategies for seamlessly integrating functional training into traditional strength programs. Sample hybrid strength programs are also provided.

Chapter 8 expands on the programming principles introduced in chapter 7 and outlines the workings of the IHP Hybrid Training System, the Three-Tier Integration System (3TIS). You will learn how 3TIS integrates functional exercises within the traditional training model, offering the most powerful training programing available today. The functional warm-up, build-up, and unloading are illustrated to guide you through the design of weekly and monthly programs. The chapter concludes with several sample workouts you can use immediately.

Chapter 9 provides 11 programs for the major sport categories. These categories classify sports that are similar in biomechanics and energy systems. For easy referencing and consistency, the exercises in these programs come from the exercises previously provided in part II.

PART I

Function and Functional Training

CHAPTER 1

Functional Training Defined

Functional training exploded onto the scene 20 years ago, yet the term is still used to describe just about any training that is not bodybuilding. This chapter lays the groundwork for this training method by providing basic definitions and applied concepts. The applied approach taken in this first chapter will enhance your understanding of what functional training is and how to use it to enhance performance.

What Is Functional Strength?

Strength training has been debated as hotly as any other topic in the strength and conditioning field. One reason for the hot discussion is that there are several types of strength and several ways to evaluate them. Let's take a closer look at each type.

Absolute strength is the most common type of strength that people talk about. Absolute strength is the greatest amount of weight an athlete can lift. Sometimes absolute strength is what you want. For example, weightlifting competitors need maximum absolute strength in all of their lifts for successful competition.

Relative strength is an athlete's absolute strength divided by body weight, and it is also a popular form of strength within the athletic arena. Relative strength is where the term *pound per pound* comes from. This type of strength is crucial for athletes who compete in weight-class sports. The strongest person in a weight class has the strength advantage every athlete is looking for.

Functional strength is the amount of strength an athlete can use on the field, and it's the most important strength to develop for sports that are not weightlifting related. However, it can be challenging to train, monitor, and communicate about functional strength. Functional training is popular within the sport world and obviously aims at developing functional strength, though it is often confused with sport-specific training.

Sport-specific training includes many exercises that are appropriate during the later phase of training when specific strength is developed. It attempts to rehearse the sport skill with some light resistance. Examples of sport-specific drills include resisted running with a band, pushing a tackling or blocking sled, and swinging a heavy bat. Functional training, on the other hand, focuses on the application of functional strength to a sport skill (i.e., the coordination of various muscle systems), not necessarily the sport skill itself. For example, a single-leg stability ball (SB) bridge improves running by enhancing hip extension, but it does not involve running the way that resisted running does. Similarly, a band or cable press can develop the force generation pattern associated with blocking without actually hitting the blocking sled. Finally, short band rotations and low-to-high cable chops develop the hip power and core stiffness necessary for bat speed, but they do not feature the complete batting motion. In essence, functional strength allows an athlete to apply strength to a sport skill. It's the best and most progressive way to improve athletic performance without actually doing a sport-specific drill or exercise.

Almost all strength and conditioning coaches now claim to do functional training. However, finding qualified strength professionals who are well versed in this method of training is difficult.

The only drawback to functional strength is that it is trained and evaluated with movement quality, not a load or number. Whereas a lift (e.g., bench press) is trained with a specific load and has a number for evaluating strength, a single-leg contralateral-arm (CLA) anterior reach uses a certain quality of movement and light training load to develop and evaluate single-leg stability. The subjective nature of functional strength presents a challenge when designing functional training programs and communicating about the development of functional strength.

Why Functional Training?

Functional training has become a hot topic and a popular training approach. In spite of a lack of specific research or clear definitions and a fair amount of controversy surrounding its methods, functional training is everywhere. Dozens of books have been written on the topic, and you can't attend a fitness conference or go to a sport training camp without seeing the functional training revolution. So, what makes this training method so effective and popular? The answers are simple, as we'll discuss in this section.

Little Space, Little Equipment, and Little Time

Nearly any traditional gym features thousands of square feet filled with hundreds of pieces of equipment that cost hundreds of thousands of dollars. In stark contrast, functional training gyms have lots of room with only some basic equipment around the perimeter. Functional training is about movement, not equipment. Therefore, a set of dumbbells, some medicine balls, a few hurdles, some bands, and a few stability balls can allow anyone to turn a room, a parking lot, or an athletic field into a functional training area. The low cost of equipment is another major advantage of functional training. With a few hundred dollars and a duffle bag, a coach can train a single athlete or an entire team anywhere, anytime.

Time is as scarce as money these days; everyone has busy schedules filled with responsibilities. Therefore, being able to train anywhere and at any time allows the athlete and coach to be effective where many can't. Functional training circuits are extremely effective in keeping an athlete or a team in tip-top shape, especially in season and while traveling. For example, you can take the 15 to 40 minutes spent traveling to and from a training facility and spend it training anywhere. You can perform 15- to 20-minute individual and team workouts in a parking lot, dorm hallway, gymnasium, or hotel room at any time of day or night. (See chapters 7, 8, and 9 for examples of these programs.)

Strength Without Size

A great characteristic of neuromuscular adaptation is that you can get stronger without getting bigger or heavier. This is a huge advantage for athletes who are in weight-class sports or sports where weight gain may create a disadvantage. The coordination between muscles and muscle systems also allows the body to spread the load through multiple muscle systems. This distribution of work creates less stress on any one muscle, reducing the need for a specific muscle to adapt and get bigger. With functional training, no single muscle screams; instead the entire body sings. That is the essence of athleticism.

Performance Benefits

Considering the benefits of functional training as well as its specificity-driven philosophy, it doesn't take a vivid imagination to figure out its performance benefits. Functional training can focus on and improve any sport skill. The single-leg exercise that addresses locomotion teaches the hamstrings and glutes to extend the hips and stabilize the body, increasing running speed, boosting cutting ability in field sports, and improving single-leg jumping in court sports. The level-change exercises that target jumping and lifting improve two-leg vertical jump height as well as lifting mechanics. The pushing and pulling exercises enhance punching, pushing, swimming, and throwing. Finally, the rotational exercises improve swinging, changes of direction, and rotational power generation.

Myths About Functional Training

Part of the controversy and confusion surrounding functional training is due to the misrepresentation of what functional training is. There is a fine line between an exercise that is effective and an exercise that is optimal, and we need to keep our terminology consistent. At the end of the day, the principle of specificity allows us to figure out what functional training is and what it isn't. Let's go through a few of the concepts that have been misrepresented during the evolution of functional training.

Effective Versus Optimal

To simplify the concept of functional training, we must first note the difference between effective training and optimal (functional) training. Training can be effective without having optimal transfer (i.e., without being functional). For example, a novice basketball player can use knee extensions and leg curls to improve running and jumping to some degree. These two traditional exercises may be effective in enhancing the athlete's general strength needed in running and jumping, but they will not be as effective as single-leg exercises used in more comprehensive and progressive training model, such as a three-stage developmental training model that progressively develops general, special, and specific strength. For example, if a running athlete was going to organize the training in a progressive, three-stage fashion, general strength is usually developed by traditional strength exercises, such as squats, leg presses, and power cleans. Special strength is oftentimes developed by functional exercises that more closely resemble the target activity, such as single-leg anterior reaches, single-leg squats, and single-leg stability ball bridges. Specific strength can then be developed by resisted running drills, uphill runs, and other forms of resisted running. Although this is an over simplification of the three-stage model, it provides an illustrative view of how the training becomes more specific or functional as time progresses. *Functional training is driven by the concept of specificity.* Single-leg exercises are more specific to running and jumping off a single leg than two-leg exercises, and therefore they are functional for any single-leg activity, such as a basketball player cutting and coming off a single leg for a layup.

Not All Proprioception Is Created Equal

A big word making its way into the mainstream is *proprioception*, or how body reads information from various body parts as well as the environment. This information (i.e., proprioceptive feedback) is the language the nervous system uses to figure out what is happening with the body and what move to make next. Functional training is thought to produce more proprioceptive feedback (i.e., meaningful information) than bodybuilding exercises do. For example, the leg curl uses a seated position and a fixed pattern of movement; not a lot of information is needed to execute the exercise. On the other hand, its functional counterpart, the reaching lunge, requires more coordination between the big muscle systems on the posterior aspect of the hips and uses the related muscle groups in a way that is more consistent with the running motion (i.e., teaching the hamstrings to extend the hips while controlling knee flexion). This complex coordination requires more proprioceptive feedback between the muscular system and the central nervous system. Thus, the leg curl machine is less proprioceptively enriching than the reaching lunge is because the leg curl machine stabilizes the movement and requires less proprioceptive feedback than the reaching lunge, which is not stabilized by any exterior mechanism. Coincidently, this is where the concept of unstabilized training, or stability training, comes from; the reaching lunge occurs in an unstabilized environment, requiring the body to develop the stability in order to execute the movement correctly.

Just because a high amount of neural information (proprioception) is being processed, it does not mean the information is meaningful. *The neural language of functional training must be specific to the athletic skill being targeted.* If an athletic skill requires the transfer of high forces from the ground to an implement (e.g., a bat) through stiff body segments, then that proprioceptive language must be part of the functional training to improve performance.

Balance Versus Stability

Balance training should not be confused with stability training. Unstable training environments are one of the hottest topics in functional training. For this reason we will cover this topic a bit more comprehensively than the others. Let's start with some definitions and then take the discussion from there.

As a noun, *balance* means the stability produced by the even distribution of weight on each side of the vertical axis. As a verb, it means to bring about a state of equilibrium (a state of balance between opposing forces).

Stability is the quality, state, or degree of being stable, as in the following:

  i. The strength to stand or endure; firmness

  ii. The property of a body that causes it when disturbed from a condition of equilibrium or steady motion to develop forces or moments that restore the original condition

  iii. Equipoise between contrasting, opposing, or interacting elements to resist forces tending to cause motion or change of motion

  iv. Designed so as to develop forces that restore the original condition when disturbed from a condition of equilibrium

In practical terms, balance is the act of manipulating opposing forces to create a stable state over a base of support. Stability is the control of unwanted motion to restore or maintain a position. Balance usually requires the transfer of low forces to maintain equilibrium, whereas stability usually requires the transfer of high forces to create rigidity. The best visual example of stability and balance is a pyramid (figure 1.1).

As you can see, the stable pyramid can withstand any force driven through its system; it is both strong and balanced. The balanced pyramid can't take any force except one going through its vertical axis. If you think of the body as an organic pyramid that responds to progressive multidirectional loading by getting bigger and better at maintaining stability, then you must train it while it is on its base and not its point. When the pyramid is balancing on its point, you simply cannot load it enough to create any significant adaptation.

There is nothing you can do from an unstable balanced position (e.g., one-leg balance) except stand there, balance, and wait to be pushed over by a fast-moving object. Athletes cannot transfer high forces or maintain their position in the face of hard physical contact from a narrow or small base of support; they are at the mercy of the physical forces of the environment (e.g., another athlete making physical contact). This is especially true during static conditions where athletes can't use momentum and inertia to help maintain dynamic control.

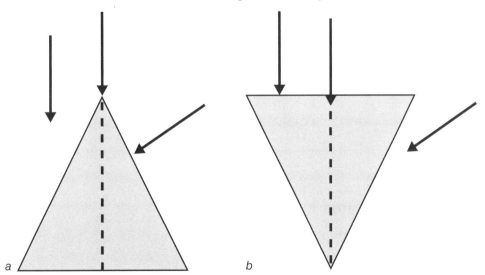

FIGURE 1.1 Stability versus balance: *(a)* This pyramid is stable and balanced. High forces can be applied to it without changing its position—certainly a quality we would want in an athlete. *(b)* This pyramid is balanced but not stable. The slightest force will topple it over—not a desirable quality in an athlete.

Functional training *must* concentrate on creating stability (i.e., super stiffness) so that proper athletic positions can be maintained and forces can be transferred through the kinetic chain. This means it must train the core in a stable state to be as stiff (rigid) as possible first and then let it move as it needs to.

Popular Functional Training Equipment

In the last two decades, the variety of functional training equipment on the market has grown to the point where figuring out what to buy and how to use it can be overwhelming. Although using a variety of equipment can add diversity to training, as well as a fun factor, most of the essential work can be done with simple equipment. There is no need for the fancy stuff if you have the right knowledge; after all, the best functional training equipment is the human body. The basic equipment discussed in this section will allow athletes to apply powerful functional training principles to stay in shape during the off-season or add a functional training component to an existing resistance workout.

Dumbbells

You can use dumbbells (abbreviated as *DB* in the exercises in this book) to load just about any functional movement you can imagine (figure 1.2). That's why they are first on the list. Dumbbells provide freedom of movement, thus requiring stabilization from each limb, which addresses upper-body imbalances in strength. The speed and loads in functional training can range from slow and heavy to explosive and light, covering all developmental stages of strength and power training.

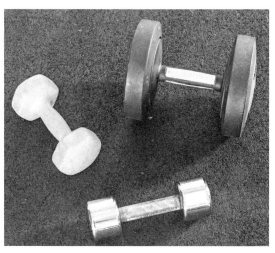

FIGURE 1.2 Dumbbells.

Dumbbells come in a variety of models, from fixed weights to selectorized or adjustable models. If you have plenty of room and would like the flexibility of training more than one person at a time, a rack of fixed-weight dumbbells is best. Functional training exercises for the most part don't use big dumbbells, so a rack of 5 to 50 pounds (2-23 kg) will serve just about anyone. If choosing a selectorized model where you can dial in or pin-load the desired weight, a 35- to 45-pound (16-20 kg) set will do the trick.

Bands and Pulleys

The next type of equipment that is a must in functional training is a good set of bands or pulleys (BP) (figure 1.3). Bands and pulleys are vital because they are the only way to provide resistance in a horizontal or diagonal direction. Due to their nonvertical loading capabilities, they are perfectly suited to provide resistance for standing exercises such as rotational chops, presses and rows, deadlifts, and lunging movements in a way no other equipment can. Single-arm exercise

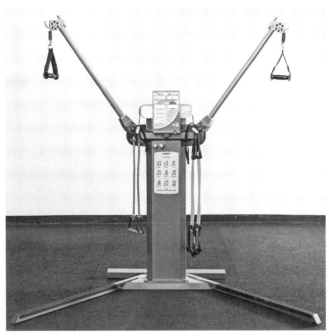

FIGURE 1.3 Bands and pulleys.

variations also can address strength imbalances between the right and left sides of the body.

Bands are more versatile than pulleys because they can be taken anywhere, can attach to a variety of structures, are inexpensive, and resist slow, heavy movements as well as light, explosive ones. A cable stack is stationary, occupies a huge space, is expensive, and is best used for heavy, slow training because light, explosive training results in a flying weight stack that eventually damages the equipment. Bands should be made of latex using the dipping process, not the extrusion process. The bands should not be continuous; they should have handles at each end and a separate attachment point to avoid wearing out the middle of the band with attachments such as nylon cords or straps.

Medicine Balls

Medicine balls (MB) (figure 1.4) come in a variety of models, from balls with handles that can be held like dumbbells to balls with ropes for swinging exercises. To keep things simple, we will deal with basic medicine balls with or without bounce capabilities. Medicine balls are excellent for loading many functional training exercises, but their best application is throws for power development.

When using a medicine ball for throws against the floor or a cement wall, a rubber model with a bounce

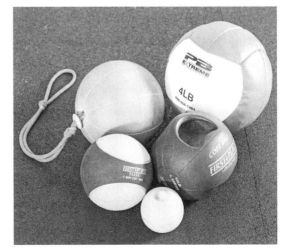

FIGURE 1.4 Medicine balls.

is the most effective. Rubber medicine balls are durable and can take the beating of power throws. If a bounce is not desired for safety reasons and the throws are going to be performed against a padded wall or floor, a synthetic-leather medicine ball is a great option. The standard weights for throws and light movement loading are in the 2- to 4-kilogram range; heavier balls are better suited for strength development and slower movements.

Stability Balls

Stability balls (SB) (figure 1.5) have come a long way. The newer models are much stronger and more burst resistant, increasing their safety. Stability balls offer a host of benefits in functional training. For example, they can support the body in certain positions that can't normally be maintained. They can also offer a measured dose of instability to training in order to facilitate greater stability at various joints.

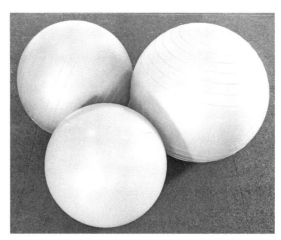

FIGURE 1.5 Stability balls.

Stability balls have been used in the past as benches for bench presses and similar exercises. However, this application has lost some favor in recent years. The dominant ideology is to use stable benches for heavy presses. Use stability balls for lighter, unstable exercises such as push-ups and to provide supportive positioning for crunches and wall slides. The most popular sizes in stability balls are 55 and 65 centimeters.

Kettlebells

Kettlebells (KB) (figure 1.6) have become popular in the functional training world. They can be used the same way as dumbbells or for more creative applications such as swings. Their extra-thick handles and unique center of mass present a gripping challenge, and they are popular with athletes looking to improve wrist stability and gripping strength. The kettlebell culture has a mind–body style and influence, creating many exercises not normally seen in the dumbbell world.

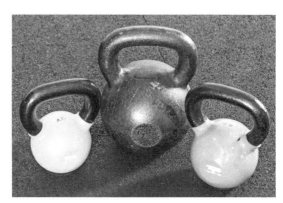

FIGURE 1.6 Kettlebells.

Kettlebell applications can range from strength exercises, such as the kettlebell overhead press, to metabolic protocols involving swings for long periods of time (2-5 minutes). This wide strength and conditioning application makes the kettlebell a worthwhile piece of equipment in your functional training toolbox. Popular weights range from 8 to 16 kilograms.

Suspension Equipment

In the last decade, suspension equipment (figure 1.7) has become popular in functional training. Before the resurgence of suspension systems, we needed an assortment of equipment to perform the various exercises that the new suspension systems easily allow. For example, in the old days, short ropes (1.5 in. [4 cm] thick and 10 ft [3 m] long) were used for recline pulls and stability balls were used for stretching exercise such as the rollout.

Today's suspension systems have stirrups and straps to secure the feet and allow users to easily adjust the strap length. They offer carabiners for easy attachment to bars and other structures, as well as expanded manuals and educational materials for suggested use. Some suspension systems, such as the *Suspended Bodyweight Training* (SBT) System, have even created their own certification and education systems for personal trainers to learn how to use them.

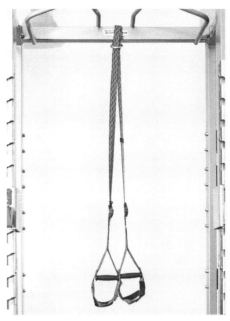

FIGURE 1.7 Suspension equipment.

Adjustable Bench

By most standards, an adjustable bench (figure 1.8) is not considered functional training equipment. However, I include it here because functional training does not exist in a vacuum; it is best used in conjunction with other training methods, including hypertrophy and strength work. Hypertrophy and strength training are beneficial, and that type of heavy training should not be done on a stability ball or other equipment not meant for heavy-loading strength applications. In addition, you can use benches for many exercise progressions that fall within the functional training realm.

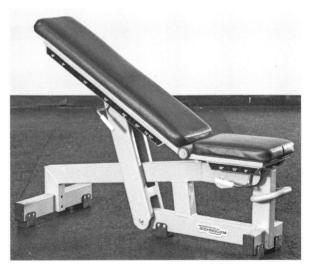

FIGURE 1.8 Adjustable bench.

The best bench is a heavy-duty one with an adjustable seat and backrest. All pressing motions, such as shoulder presses or bench presses, can be performed from a bench. Benches also can support exercises such as bent-over rows, weighted hip lifts, and various forms of sit-ups and crunches. Regardless of how the bench is used, it may be considered standard equipment in small studios, homes, or other functional training areas.

Equipment for Travel

Getting good training on the road has always been a challenge for athletes, especially during in-season travel. Whether you are a judo practitioner on the European tour, a tennis player running through a string of tournaments, or an athlete traveling for any reason that takes you away from home, traveling can ruin your conditioning if you don't find a way to get your training done. Of all the training equipment available, there is only one type that needs to be the athlete's travel partner—a good set of adjustable bands (figure 1.9).

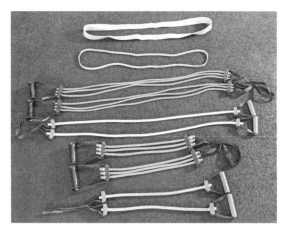

FIGURE 1.9 Adjustable bands.

A JC Predator Jr. (figure 1.10) has become my standard recommendation for the traveling athlete. I am not suggesting that a set of bands will take the place of the strength training equipment you can find in a well-equipped gym. However, resistance is resistance, and when you can't get to other equipment, the Predator Jr. can provide the right resistance to the right move-

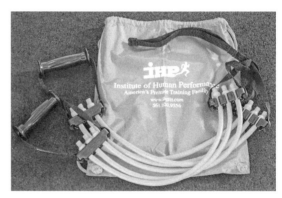

FIGURE 1.10 JC Predator Jr. and bag.

ment, allowing you to get in the training that you would otherwise miss.

Bands travel easily because of their materials, size, and easy setup. They are made of plastic and latex, which means they can quickly travel through any security point and in carry-on luggage. The Predator is small enough to fit in the pocket of a computer bag, so space is not an issue. Depending on the band model and the exercise, the setup can vary. You can anchor the band to a doorframe or simply step on the band to create resistance.

Sometimes no equipment is available when you're traveling. In these rare cases, turn to the landscape to provide equipment in the form of stairs, benches, high bars, dip bars, sand, hills, and any other structure that can be used as a training apparatus or additional resistance. The structures surrounding most hotels can create a great training environment, from bodyweight training in your room to stair exercises to training in sand.

Conclusion

This chapter has explained functional training and clarified some of the myths surrounding it. It has also made equipment recommendations that highlight the simplicity and economy of functional training. Functional training does not have to be complex or expensive to be highly effective and cutting edge. With this information, you are now ready to explore the foundations of functional training.

CHAPTER 2

Foundations of Functional Training

When discussing functional training, defining *function* is a great place to start. In its basic form, it is the action for which a person or thing is specially used or for which a thing exists—its purpose. Therefore, *functional* can be defined as

- performing a function,
- performing a duty for which a person or thing is intended, or
- a characteristic action of anything—a duty, utility, or purpose.

To define *functional training*, we must first define the function or characteristic action of the human body. In other words, what is the movement function of the human body?

Four Pillars of Human Movement

Human movement can be classified into four categories: locomotion, level changes, pushing and pulling, and rotation. These are the four pillars of human movement. The four-pillar model organizes the basic movements all bodies perform in everyday life. The model lends itself perfectly to sport in that each pillar can be associated with major sport skills, or what I refer to as the *Big Four* of sport: locomotion, level changes, throwing, and changes of direction. For the most part, if a sport requires a person to stand on both feet, the Big Four dominate the skills needed for participation in the sport. More details on the Big Four are provided later in this chapter.

Locomotion

The first pillar of human movement is *locomotion*. As bipedal animals, locomotion is our most basic biomotor skill. Everyone, especially locomotive-based athletes, should therefore consider relating all training to the human gait cycle.

Two major characteristics of locomotion are single-leg stability and rotation. Locomotion occurs one leg at a time, creating a structure that transfers forces from the ground to the rest of the body. This is called the *7-frame*, and it will be discussed in more detail later in the chapter. Rotation is a major component of locomotion that is necessary to cancel rotational force between the upper and lower body, which maintains the body alignment and balance necessary for efficient running.

Locomotion is the primary biomotor skill because it integrates all four pillars. With each stride, the center of mass moves both horizontally and vertically (i.e., level changes—pillar 2). Locomotion involves the contralateral push-and-pull movements of the upper body (i.e., pushing and pulling—pillar 3), which are essential for canceling the rotational forces generated by the lower body. The contralateral movement between the upper and lower body creates the rotational component (i.e., rotation—pillar 4) of linear locomotion that is fundamental to efficient forward movement. This integration is why there are four pillars and why they are presented in this order.

Level Changes

The second pillar of human movement involves level changes in a person's center of mass. *Level changes* are characterized by movements of the trunk or lower extremities or a combination of the two that lower or raise the center of mass. These level changes are necessary for performing many nonlocomotive tasks, such as picking up objects, getting into low positions, or getting up off the floor. With the lower body, we can perform level changes by squatting, lunging, or stepping up on or down off objects by simply flexing the ankles, knees, and hips. Therefore, the primary method of lower-body force production is made possible by the triple-extension mechanism involving the ankle, knee, and hip. The trunk of the body can also help to vertically displace the center of mass by flexing or extending the spine. Most of the time we use a combination of trunk and lower-extremity flexion to perform functional level changes (e.g., low volley in tennis, suplex in wrestling, scramble up after falling). Note that gravity, not the flexor chain of the muscular system, is responsible for the descent of the level change (i.e., total-body flexion). The extensor chain controls the speed and degree of flexion in function, and thus level-change injuries usually occur in the posterior structures of the body (e.g., Achilles tendon, hamstrings, lower back).

Pushing and Pulling

The third pillar of human movement is *pushing and pulling*. These movements involve the upper body and can displace the combined center of mass. For simplicity, we will consider a pull to be any movement that brings the elbows or hands inward or toward the main line of the body. Pulling brings things close to us to hold or carry, and it also occurs in the initial acceleration stage of throwing an object. A push is any movement that brings the elbows or hands outward or away from the main line of the body. Pushing involves activities such as pushing away an opponent or pushing off the ground to get up after a fall, and it also occurs in the latter part of throwing (i.e., late portion of acceleration and follow-through).

Pushing and pulling are also part of our reflex and biomechanical systems. Our bodies are neurologically cross wired; a reflex causes one limb to flex as the contralateral limb extends. This phenomenon can be seen in many explosive actions, such as throwing, swimming, and running. For example, in sport skills such as punching and throwing, the left elbow flexes as the right arm extends and comes through to punch or to throw a ball. By creating short lever arms, the body increases its rotational speed (much like a figure skater rotates faster as the arms come in toward the main line of the body). In running, we can see this reflex and matching lever arms between the upper and lower body. When the left arm is behind the body with the elbow flexed (short lever arm), the right leg is also up and flexed (short lever arm). Simultaneously, the right arm is more extended while the left leg is more extended and pushing off the ground.

Rotation

The neural cross wiring just described leads us to the last and most important pillar of human movement: *rotation.* This pillar is responsible for what replays in sport are usually made out of—rotational power! It's the most important pillar because many physical movements in sport are explosive and involve the transverse plane (i.e., the plane of movement where rotation takes place).

A quick look at the muscular system shows how heavily human movement relies on rotation. In their 1970 book *Kinesiology*, Gene A. Logan and Wayne C. McKinney describe the serape effect.[1] The authors do a fantastic job explaining how and why the body uses this muscular cross wiring to provide rotational power. If you want to see the serape effect at work, stand in front of a mirror wearing a loose T-shirt. Go through a throwing motion and freeze at the top of the throw. Or, simply march in place. Watch how the shirt wrinkles. How do the core muscles load up during throwing or running? Diagonally!

Pull out an anatomy book and look at the core musculature. You will see that most of the core musculature is in a diagonal or horizontal orientation. Of the major muscles in the core (i.e., major muscles attached to the trunk, above the ischial tuberosity, and below the superior aspect of the sternum), almost 90 percent are oriented either diagonally or horizontally and have rotation as one of their major functions. Table 2.1 provides a rough organization of core muscles and their basic orientation, which clearly illustrates the rotational nature of the body.

Big Four Sport Skills

The four most common movement categories—the Big Four—in sport are locomotion, level changes, pushing and pulling (throwing, pushing away, and holding objects), and rotation (changes of direction). They are at the heart of most ground-based sports (i.e., sports performed from the standing position) and are almost identical to the four pillars of human movement. The four pillars describe the biomechanical functions of the body that no sport can violate; therefore, the Big Four must mirror the four pillars. Bipedal (i.e., two-leg) locomotion will always be the way we get from point A to point B. Level changes will always dictate the loading mechanism for jumping, picking up objects, and getting into low athletic positions. Pushing and pulling are natural movements that occur often. Table 2.2 shows the Big Four, their basic motions, and sport-specific activities that fall into each category.

---

[1] Logan, G., and W. McKinney. 1970. The serape effect. In *Anatomical kinesiology*, 3rd ed., ed. A. Lockhart, 287-302. Dubuque, IA: Brown.

TABLE 2.1 Core Muscles and Their Orientation

DORSAL		
Muscle	**Nonvertical**	**Vertical**
Trapezius	✓	
Rhomboid	✓	
Latissimus dorsi	✓	
Serratus posterior	✓	
Erector spinae		✓
Quadratus lumborum	✓	
Gluteus maximus	✓	
Gluteus medius	✓	
Tensor fasciae latae		✓
Rotators of the hip (6)	✓	

VENTRAL		
Muscle	**Nonvertical**	**Vertical**
Pectoralis major	✓	
Pectoralis minor	✓	
Serratus anterior	✓	
External oblique	✓	
Internal oblique	✓	
Rectus abdominis		✓
Transversus abdominis	✓	
Psoas	✓	
Iliacus	✓	
Sartorius	✓	
Rectus femoris		✓
Adductors (3)	✓	
Pectineus	✓	
Gracilis	✓	
Total	28 pairs = 56	4 pairs = 8
% of rotational muscles	87.5%	12.5%

As mentioned, the Big Four sport movements are described by the four pillars of human movement. They are also all powered by a series of muscles discussed later in this chapter, the anterior and posterior serape. Relating the major movements in sport to the four pillars and then developing a biomechanical model to train the movements creates a simple yet powerful way of designing functional

TABLE 2.2 Motions and Sample Activities of the Big Four Sport Skills

Sport skill	Basic motion	Sample sport-specific activities
Locomotion	Any locomotive movement that takes the body from point A to point B	All walking, jogging, running, shuffling, skipping, and jumping taking off from a single leg
Level changes	Flexion and extension of the legs or core that raises or lowers the body's center of mass, including lifting from the ground	Lowering the body to field a low grounder in baseball, hitting a low volley in tennis, getting up after falling, sprawling and lifting an opponent in wrestling, and lowering the center of mass to decelerate
Pushing and pulling (throwing, pushing away, and holding objects)	Launching an implement with one hand, usually requiring the other arm to go in the opposite direction; pushing away and holding on to objects may require one or both limbs to work in a coordinated fashion	Throwing in baseball, serving in tennis, spiking in volleyball, and throwing a javelin
Rotation (changes of direction)	Any movement that requires planting one leg and rotating the hips and shoulders, including swinging an implement	Changing locomotive direction in all sports, batting, golfing, throwing a hammer, swimming, and aerial rotations

training programs for sport. Now, let's look at the Big Four and how they relate to the four pillars in more specific terms.

Sport Locomotion

In ground-based sports, locomotion (running) is arguably the most important skill needed for success. Running speed and agility are at the top of the wish list when athletes come to a strength and conditioning coach. This is one reason why locomotion is the first of the four pillars of human movement and involves all the other pillars.

Locomotion is any action that uses alternating leg movements to move the body from point A to point B. During locomotion, a single foot is planted on the ground, and that ground contact transfers energy to move the hips in an intended direction. The hips travel over the planted foot, the other foot is planted on the ground, and the cycle continues. Whether an athlete is running to first base, shuffling to get into position around a basketball pick, or changing directions on a tennis court, sport locomotion eventually puts the body's weight on a single leg, and that is one of the fundamental features we need to see, understand, and train. Transferring high forces through a single leg is the key feature of the first pillar and all sport locomotion. Let's look at this single-leg phenomenon so we can better understand its importance and how to train it.

Most traditional methods of improving running performance use some form of two-legged strength training, such as squats, deadlifts, and leg presses. Although these exercises will improve locomotion, they are not specific to sport skills. When training for strength using two-leg exercises, the athlete uses the

A-frame. In architecture, the A-frame is a structure that allows buildings to be constructed with many floors stacked on top of each other. Because of its stability, the A-frame is the position used for the heaviest lifts, such as squats (figure 2.1a).

Although the squat is a good general exercise, it doesn't provide optimal carryover to running when compared with single-leg exercises such as the single-leg squat. Unlike the A-frame of a two-leg squat, the single-leg squat uses the 7-frame (figure 2.1b).

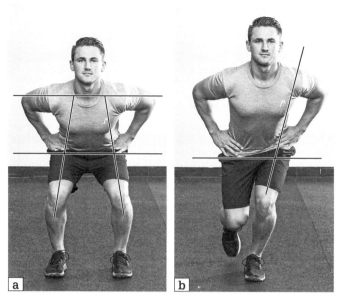

FIGURE 2.1 Two versions of the squat: *(a)* A two-legged squat uses the A-frame position; *(b)* a single-leg squat uses the 7-frame position.

The 7-frame requires superior stability of the ground-based hip when compared with the A-frame. Any instability of the ground-based hip results in an inhibitory process that shuts down the body's ability to produce a force (i.e., strength) that would put the unstable hip in danger. Obviously, the negative aspect of protecting the hip with an inhibitory response is that it reduces the power provided by the hip and slows down the locomotive process. Therefore, training the 7-frame not only strengthens single-hip stability but also reduces the inhibitory response that a weak hip would experience.

Locomotion has additional features involving the coordination of the contralateral upper and lower limbs. We will discuss these in more detail later in this chapter.

Many popular functional training exercises for locomotion are simple movements with big returns. Some of the exercises already mentioned in this book are some of my favorites, including the single-leg anterior reach, the single-leg squat, and the single-leg SB bridge. These three exercises are the staples of my running program. Two additional exercises are the single-leg lateral wall slide and the wall march. These six exercises make a great at-home running program and are covered in more details in chapters 3 through 5. Table 2.3 shows an example of how you can develop sport locomotion at home or in a gym.

Level Changes

Level changes occur when an athlete performs a countermovement before a jump, falls and gets up, goes for a ball that is close to the ground, lifts an opponent or object, changes levels in any combat sport, or simply changes directions. This crucial athletic skill is seen in just about all ground-based sports, which is why it is the second pillar of human movement. Let's look at the mechanics of level changes so we can better understand how they happen and how to train them functionally.

TABLE 2.3 Home or Gym Functional Training Program for Running

MONDAY AND THURSDAY		TUESDAY AND FRIDAY	
Exercise	**Sets and reps**	**Exercise**	**Sets and reps**
Single-leg CLA anterior reach	2 or 3 × 10	Single-leg squat	2 or 3 × 10
SB single-leg lateral wall slide (inside leg)	2 or 3 × 10	SB bridge (single leg)	2 or 3 × 10
45-degree wall march or run	2 or 3 × 10-20 (or 10-20 sec)	SB single-leg lateral wall slide (outside leg)	2 or 3 × 10

Level changes require flexion of the legs, hips, and even the spine to varying degrees to lower the body's center of mass. Even when significant knee flexion is involved, the hips (i.e., the center of the posterior core) do most of the work to control level changes in sport. Relying on the posterior side of the core to do the heavy lifting makes sense because it involves the huge muscle groups of the hamstrings, glutes, and paraspinal muscles. I affectionately call these three muscle groups the *three amigos.* Most injuries in noncontact sports involve these muscles in one way or another, so training them not only makes sense for performance, it also makes sense for injury prevention.

In most sports, level changes use two bases of support (figure 2.2): the parallel stance and the staggered stance. Both bases of support are used when getting up off the ground, lowering the body to get to an object, and lifting the body or an object. A basketball player uses the parallel stance to perform the level change needed to set up a jump shot. A baseball catcher may also use the parallel stance in his low stationary position to provide the stability needed before reacting to a runner trying to steal a base. During some athletic skills, such as a wrestling suplex, the parallel stance is used to deadlift an opponent off the mat. During some lifting skills, athletes also use their arms to hold on to opponents (objects), bringing in the pulling motion that is part of the third pillar.

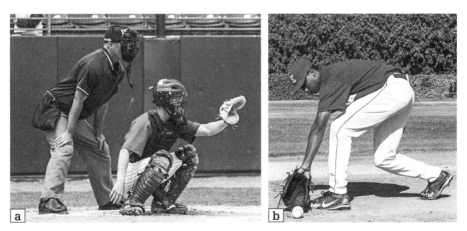

FIGURE 2.2 Level changes occur with two bases of support. In baseball, *(a)* a catcher uses a parallel stance to provide the stability needed to react to a wild pitch or a runner trying to steal, but *(b)* an infielder uses a staggered stance to quickly field and throw a low grounder.

Level changes performed from the staggered stance are quite different from their parallel-stance counterparts. These movements require more finesse and are used with more surgical precision. Low volleys in tennis are a perfect example of the fast level changes of the combined reaching for a ball and decelerating locomotion (running). Infielders in baseball also need to field fast-moving low grounders that require the staggered stance. The staggered-stance level change not only offers fast level changes, it also offers the ability to execute a fast change of direction so that a player can get back in the game or continue a play.

Regardless of the timing used by the upper and lower body, one thing stands out when we observe the staggered-stance level change: the single-leg and single-hip dominance of the 7-frame. Although both feet may be on the ground in the staggered stance, one side takes most of the load when decelerating or changing directions. This single-side dominance and the asymmetrical loading that accompanies it are not addressed in traditional two-leg training methods. It is this specificity that functional training addresses so effectively.

Once we analyze the two positions used for level changes in most sports, we can use the principle of specificity to train them. Traditional strength training focuses on the parallel stance and the symmetrical loading of the A-frame. Exercises such as deadlifts, good mornings, squats, and Olympic lifts all address the parallel-stance level change. These traditional exercises are effective in developing basic strength and can be part of a comprehensive, year-round strength and conditioning program. However, a lack of time, facilities, money, coaching skills, and athletic ability may prevent these traditional training methods from being used. In these cases, a more functional approach to training can be a great alternative. Kettlebell swings, wood chops, parallel-stance compound rows, and SB reverse hyperextensions are all excellent options for developing the posterior musculature and improving level changes from the parallel stance.

Considering how often the staggered stance appears in sport, the single-leg dominance of the staggered-stance level change has not been trained with as much frequency and focus as it should be. Traditionally, two-leg, symmetrically loaded exercises have been used to train all level changes. This type of oversight allowed functional training to emerge as an alternative system of training. Functional training acknowledges the obvious position of the staggered stance and trains it with single-leg and staggered-stance exercises focused on hip hinging. This attention to biomechanical specificity has yielded incredible results in a short time with simple exercises and without expensive and bulky equipment. Exercises such as the BP staggered-stance CLA compound row, BP staggered-stance CLA deadlift, and the single-leg 45-degree back extension are among the most effective exercises used to develop fast level changes from the staggered stance. Table 2.4 shows an example of an easy level-change program that can be used twice per week for about 30 minutes each session.

Pushing and Pulling (Throwing)

Just like locomotion in sport, let's take throwing as an example. If we were to observe a pitcher launching a 100 miles-per-hour (161 kph) fastball, we would see that he lunges from one leg to the other, changes his level, pulls and pushes with his arms, and rotates his body. This integration of all four pillars is common in many sport activities, which is why it is such a powerful model to use for analysis and exercise design. Even when looking at other sport skills within the throwing

TABLE 2.4 Home or Gym Functional Training Program for Level Changes

PARALLEL STANCE		STAGGERED STANCE	
Exercise	Sets and reps	Exercise	Sets and reps
Barbell deadlift	3 × 10	BP staggered-stance CLA compound row	3 × 10 per leg
BP compound row	3 × 10	BP staggered-stance CLA deadlift	3 × 10 per leg
SB reverse hyperextension	3 × 10	Single-leg 45-degree back extension	3 × 10 per leg

category, such as an overhead serve in tennis or a spike in volleyball, all four pillars are represented.

The force-generation patterns of throwing are similar to running and changing direction in that they are powered by diagonal patterns of force generation—the power highways. As you can see in figure 2.3, a right-handed pitcher sends the ball flying toward the catcher by using a diagonal pattern of force generation that crosses the back of the body (i.e., right hip to left shoulder during the windup and cocking phases) and the front of the body (i.e., the right shoulder to the left hip during the acceleration phase). The pitcher uses locomotion to push off and take the step to home plate after the cocking phase, and he uses a level change when opening the stance, push and pull to actually throw the ball, and rotation while everything is going on during the acceleration and follow-through phases. This is how all four pillars are used to throw a ball.

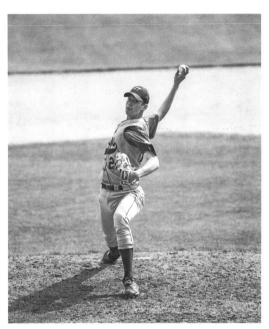

FIGURE 2.3 Acceleration of a pitch. Although the forward thrust of a right-handed pitcher is provided by the diagonal posterior musculature going from the right hip to the left shoulder, the acceleration of the ball is powered by the muscles oriented diagonally in front of the body from the right shoulder to the left hip: right serratus anterior, right external oblique, left internal oblique, and left hip flexors and adductors.

You will find similar integration of all pillars in most overhead activities that involve propelling something forward.

Once the pitch has been launched, a similar diagonal pattern decelerates the pitching action across the backside of the body (figure 2.4). The deceleration position of a pitcher is powered by the muscles oriented diagonally in the back of the body from the left hip to the right shoulder: left hamstrings, left glutes, and right latissimus dorsi. If you look closely at pictures of any motion, you will often see the clothing stretch in the direction the forces are generated. This is a great tool for determining the muscles that align themselves with a motion. We provide more information on this diagonal pattern later in this chapter when we discuss the serape and highways of power.

One big mistake to avoid when analyzing the pitching or serving motion is looking where injuries mostly occur—the shoulder. If you look at the shoulder of a pitcher during the pitching motion or a tennis player during the serving motion, you will see an incredible amount of rotation (figure 2.5). When the shoulder gets injured, the normal course of action is rest, ice, and eventually rotator cuff exercises. However, this traditional approach to analyzing and training throwers needs to be reevaluated. This is not the way to train the rotators of the shoulder to move through the range and at the speed used in sport.

What accelerates and decelerates the arm in throwing or serving motions is not the shoulder but rather the core. The body acts like a bow, with the strong portion that is generating the power located right in the middle (the core). This area must be trained with big movements so the front of the body learns to accelerate the throwing motion and the back of the body learns to decelerate it.

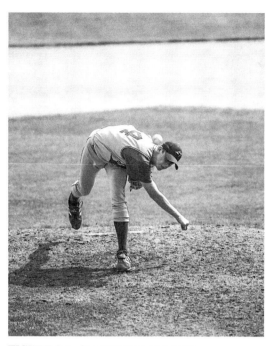

FIGURE 2.4   Deceleration of a pitch.

In order to train the throwing acceleration and deceleration components in a more functional manner, you have to consider both phases of throwing. Most athletes and coaches concern themselves with the acceleration component, but that is similar to adding more horsepower to a car with weak brakes. The BP staggered-stance CLA press and X-up are examples of easy exercises that provide the diagonal core training needed to improve throwing speed and prevent injury.

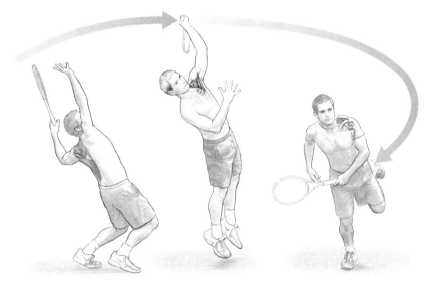

FIGURE 2.5   Shoulder rotation during the tennis serve.

Adapted, by permission, from E.P. Roetert and M.S. Kovacs, 2011, *Tennis anatomy* (Champaign, IL: Human Kinetics), 26.

These exercises teach the core to do the majority of the work so the shoulder and wrist don't have to. Not only does this approach provide more power and speed, it keeps the small joints happy and less susceptible to injury.

The deceleration phase of throwing is possibly more important than the acceleration phase. Many of the injuries in throwing occur on the backside of the body. The cool thing about the deceleration of the throwing motion is that it is the same as locomotion and level changes because it involves both of them. Exercises such as the SB reverse hyperextensions and KB single-arm swing are excellent to develop deceleration capabilities. To these two exercises you can add more specific exercises, such as the single-leg CLA anterior reach, BP staggered-stance CLA compound row, and DB or KB front reaching lunge.

You can easily perform a weekly functional training throwing program out of the home or at any gym with simple, inexpensive equipment. Table 2.5 illustrates such a program.

TABLE 2.5 Home or Gym Functional Training Program for Throwing

MONDAY AND THURSDAY (ACCELERATION DAY)		TUESDAY AND FRIDAY (DECELERATION DAY)	
Exercise	Sets and reps	Exercise	Sets and reps
Plank	2 or 3 × 10	Single-leg CLA anterior reach	2 or 3 × 10
X-up	2 or 3 × 10	BP compound row	2 or 3 × 10
BP staggered-stance press	2 or 3 × 10 per arm	DB or KB front reaching lunge	2 or 3 × 10 per leg

Rotation (Changes of Direction)

Without a doubt, rotation (changes of direction and swinging implements) are the most important movement skill of the Big Four. Changes of direction, including implement swings, are featured in almost all sports, and they are often behind the great replays we see in sport. Whether a running back fakes out a linebacker or a batter hits a home run, the rotational ability needed to load the body in one direction and explosively change directions is often a defining moment in sport (figure 2.6). Rotation is the essence of this skill, and it is also the fourth pillar of human movement, the thread that interconnects all other pillars.

Change of direction and its rotational component are fundamental to human movement, especially power generation.

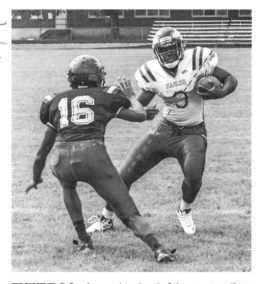

FIGURE 2.6 A running back fakes out a linebacker. This change of direction is loaded by the diagonal musculature of the back: the big latissimus dorsi and the opposite glutes and hamstrings.

The rotational component has many faces. For example, if you analyze human locomotion, you quickly realize the upper body moves in opposition to the lower body; that is, the right arm comes forward at the same time the left leg does. If you study the pitching motion of a right-handed pitcher, you will see the left leg and right arm come together in the windup and then separate as the pitcher steps (strides) toward home plate into the cocking phase. As the hips turn to home plate to begin to accelerate the ball, the right arm comes toward the left leg again during the follow-through. Similarly, a batter or a golfer separates the right shoulder from the left leg during the backswing and stride (figure 2.7). Then as the hips rotate and the bat or club comes through the impact zone, the right shoulder comes toward the left hip.

All of these examples have a few things in common:

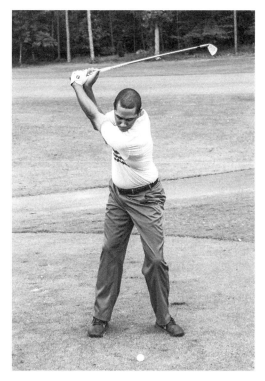

FIGURE 2.7 The backswing in golf. The right-handed golf swing is loaded by the posterior and diagonal musculature of the back (i.e., right hamstring, right glutes, left latissimus dorsi) and the opposite musculature in the front (i.e., left hip flexors and adductor complex, left internal oblique, right external oblique, right serratus anterior).

- Most of the changes of direction occur off a fixed point on the ground.
- They need a dominant point-of-ground contact (usually single-leg dominant) in order to push in a given direction.
- After the initial leg drive, all changes of direction are initiated by a rotational hip movement that is followed by the shoulders.
- The pattern of force generation in these changes of direction is diagonal, connecting one hip to the opposite shoulder through the front and back of the body.
- Changing direction involves the deceleration of a force and immediate acceleration of another force in another direction.
- The core (the area between the chest and thighs) is the bridge that transfers the power expressed in the change of direction.

These topics will be covered in more detail later in this chapter when we discuss the highways of sport power.

From our discussion on the diagonal and rotational nature of changes of direction, it is obvious that in order to train this popular sport movement in a functional manner, you have to train rotational and diagonal movements. Even movements that load a single extremity (e.g., single-arm press, single-arm row) can feature enough of a rotational component to provide excellent functional training for changes of direction. Many of the lower-body exercises already mentioned, such as the single-leg CLA anterior reach and the reaching lunge, can also provide excellent training for changes of direction. However, if we consider the principle of specificity, we can easily see that adding more lateral and rotational training can further improve functional training for sports that feature lateral changes in direction. For example, exercises such as the lateral reaching lunge, MB diagonal chop, BP short rotation, and diagonal BP chop provide more targeted rotational training that is sure to make you faster and add rotational power to sport skills that involve swinging. Table 2.6 provides a sure-bet way to improve locomotive changes of direction as well as swinging power.

The Big Four offer a way to associate the major sport movements with the four pillars and create functional training programs based on the principle of specificity. Biomechanics can be a complicated subject, but when analyzed in a logical and sport-specific manner, exercise design and programming become easier to implement using the simple programs offered in this book. Therein lies the strength of the Big Four!

TABLE 2.6 Supporting Exercises for Changes of Direction (Including Swings)

LOCOMOTIVE CHANGES OF DIRECTION		SWINGING	
Exercise	Sets and reps	Exercise	Sets and reps
DB or KB lateral reaching lunge	3 × 10	BP short rotation (10 to 2 o'clock)	3 × 10 per leg
SB single-leg lateral wall slide	3 × 10	BP low-to-high chop	3 × 10 per leg
MB short diagonal chop	3 × 10	BP high-to-low chop	3 × 10 per leg

Athletic Environment

The powerful movement models discussed up to now allow athletic expression due to the environment that athletics occur in. This environment has been rarely acknowledged, much less used to define and enhance functional training. Most sports take place on land (i.e., require ground contact during the execution of skills), but some sports feature eclectic physical environments. For instance, the strokes in swimming occur in water and the aerial maneuvers in diving occur in air.

Dryland strength training for sports not dominated by ground contact still occurs on land. If your strength training takes place on land, then the operational environment of ground-based function automatically dominates training and must be taken into account. Understanding the properties that affect the ground-based training environment will help you maximize the functional training principles explained throughout this book.

Gravity

The most striking and consistent component of our operational environment is gravity. Gravity affects all objects on earth by influencing them with a downward force (i.e., acceleration). This downward force provides a few important tools used in practically all sports and ground-based training.

First, the pull of gravity loads muscle systems. For example, if you are going to jump, you automatically relax your legs and hips, allowing gravity to quickly flex your body and load the extensor muscles so you can jump with more power. The flexing did not cost the body any energy due to the pull of gravity, and the speed at which gravity pulls the body down can even elicit reflexes (e.g., myostatic reflex) in some plyometric exercises, such as depth jumps. If you want to see the absence or reduction of gravity, look at how slowly astronauts move in space. Can you imagine playing a sport on the moon? It would take forever and have no power.

Gravity also allows us to simultaneously load joints in three planes of motion. During his Chain Reaction seminar (1995), Gary Gray referred to this loading mechanism as *multiplane joint motion*, or triplanar loading. For example, when a right-handed golfer allows gravity to act on the right hip during the backswing, the hip flexes in the sagittal plane, adducts in the frontal plane, and internally loads in the transverse plane. This triplanar loading of the hip provides the big power you see in the drive. With few exceptions, all major joints in the body can load in a triplanar fashion, making the human body and gravity strong allies in power generation.

Triplanar loading puts various body segments in the best biomechanical position to generate power and create the next physical element, momentum. Functional training has to reflect this use of gravity to load muscles as well as to elicit reflexes. Exercises such as various jumps, low-to-high cable rotations, and medicine ball throws can be of great use in learning how to use gravity to create power.

Momentum

Momentum is one of the most visible qualities in sport and the one that dominates power. It is used to load muscle and to move efficiently through big ranges of motion. For example, momentum is used in plyometric training to load muscles for a more forceful contraction. Momentum is also responsible for the long ranges traveled by implements, objects, and body parts using little if any muscular contraction; think of Michael Jordan's single-leg takeoffs during his winning dunk performances. The momentum created by the backswing is what provides the power of a batting or golf swing.

Momentum is the product of an object's mass and speed; the faster an object moves or the larger it is, the more momentum it will have. In real life, mass usually stays constant. An athlete's body weight, a bat, a ball, a glove, and a racket stay the same weight. In these cases the factor that increases momentum is speed, which is why they say speed kills. Acceleration is the increase in speed, and it is one of the most sought-after qualities in sport. On the other hand, a reduction in momentum is often referred to as *deceleration*. As previously mentioned, deceleration is as important as acceleration when it comes to athletic performance. Both acceleration and deceleration are dynamic qualities that involve strength and speed, and the functional training for sport should reflect this. Exercises such as skips, skaters, and medicine ball throws are great for teaching an athlete how to manipulate momentum and work simultaneously on the strength and speed components.

Ground Reaction Forces

Another characteristic of our operational environment is the ground-based nature of force production. For the most part, everything we prepare for requires us to generate forces from the ground up. Whether we are swinging a bat, picking up an opponent in a combat sport, or blocking a defensive tackle in football, the force generated for the activity is determined by the athlete's ability to transfer forces to and from the ground via a solid foot contact and ground reaction forces.

Isaac Newton explains the reason for this in his third law of motion, the law of action and reaction. It states that for every action, there is always an opposed and equal reaction. This means that when you are standing and applying forces to the ground, the ground provides an equal amount of force back. Therefore, when you plant your foot on the ground during the plant phase of running, the ground provides the same amount of force back to you, propelling your hips in the intended direction.

Ground reaction forces also influence our approach to balance training and how we use unstable surfaces. Although balance training may be effective in keeping neurological pathways open and neural communication flowing, balance (i.e., unstable) training does not provide the stability needed to transmit high forces via solid foot contact with the ground, as is required in all ground-based sports. It is impossible to react with the ground when something soft or unstable is between the ground and the body! Because we need to react with the ground in order to transmit force, we must reevaluate the use of balance training for producing and transmitting power. Our recommendation is simple: Plant your feet on the ground and move heavy stuff as fast as you can in all directions!

Ground reaction forces are important in all sports, even those such as swimming. As previously mentioned, even if the sport itself does not rely much on ground contact, the strength training in a gym is mostly all ground based. Therefore, the effectiveness of strength development in a gym is based on ground contact and reaction.

Three Planes of Motion

The last element of the operational environment is its three-dimensional nature. Every day we operate in an environment that has 360 degrees of movement capability. This freedom of movement provides enormous strength and power capabilities through triplanar loading.

Because most, if not all, athletic movement takes place in a multiplanar environment, it only makes sense to train consistently in that environment. We must train in a manner that involves all three planes of motion if we are going to prepare for the multiplanar environment of sport. The three planes of motion provide many advantages. For example, 360 degrees of movement allows muscles to load in three planes of motion simultaneously. However, this incredible benefit must also be stabilized through all three planes, which is called *triplanar stability*. The lack of triplanar stability is a key drawback of traditional training, especially machine-based training, but it is a key attribute developed by functional training.

Highways of Sport Power

The body connects its major muscle systems to create highways of power in the most common sport movements. Creating a map of these highways of power provides a new training model that encompasses all of the directions the body moves in and a training model that corresponds to those directions—my training octagon.

Body as the Ultimate Bow: Direction of Athletic Force Production

One of the simplest ways to illustrate how the body generates power is to compare it to a bow. Everyone knows that in order to load a bow, you must first bend the bow (figure 2.8*a*). We also know that the strongest and stiffest part of the bow is the center, or the core.

For example, a tennis player bends his body back to serve a ball (figure 2.8*b*). This backward bending loads the front bow of the body. Like the bow, the tennis player gets his power from his center. This analogy reveals the specificity of simple exercises, such as the BP swim and the MB overhead slam. These two exercises can train the front bow of the body and improve any overhead throwing activity.

Staying with the bow analogy, the body also bends to load the back bow. The back bow can load and provide the power for all level changes (e.g., jumping, getting up off the ground, lifting objects). For example, a swimmer or sprinter bends (flexes) her entire back musculature to load the back bow for pushing off the starting blocks and for turning off the wall. Likewise, a wrestler picks up an opponent with the core muscles of the back bow.

This visual allows us to appreciate the specificity of general strength exercises, such as the deadlift, and more specific functional exercises, such as the KB single-arm swing and the MB reverse scoop throw. The front and back bow not only accelerate flexion and extension, they also work in opposition to each other in a cooperative way, as we'll see when we look at their diagonal components.

Anterior and Posterior Serape

Expanding on the bow analogy and the diagonal loading of the core, we can view the body as a series of bows connected as a ribbon or scarf. This diagonal config-

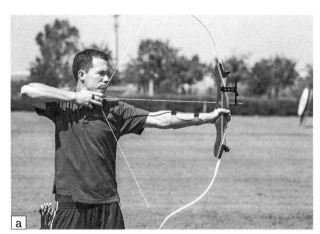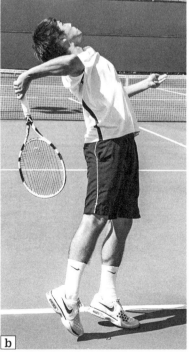

FIGURE 2.8 *(a)* The archer bends the bow in order to load it. *(b)* The tennis player bends the body in order to create power when serving.

uration is called the *anterior serape* (figure 2.9) and the *posterior serape* (figure 2.10). This biomechanical system is extremely important in sport, and understanding it will serve us well in learning how the body moves and how to train it.

The anterior serape connects the right shoulder to the left leg and the left shoulder to the right leg along the front of the body. To complete the ribbon figure, each shoulder is posteriorly connected to the spine by way of the scapulae. In direct opposition, the posterior serape connects the right shoulder to the left leg and the left shoulder to the right leg along the backside of the body. To complete the ribbon figure, each shoulder is connected anteriorly to the sternum by the pectorals (chest muscles). It may seem contradictory to have an anterior muscular system connected by posterior musculature and a posterior muscular system connected by anterior musculature, but this configuration makes perfect sense when you think about similar examples in everyday life. A belt has to come around the back to secure the front of the garment, a scarf wraps around the back to hold the front in place, and a coat has to have a back to hold the front in place. The anterior and posterior serapes work in a coordinated agonist and antagonist fashion; whatever the anterior serape accelerates, the posterior serape decelerates, and vice versa.

To bring the serape to life, let's use the previous example of the right-handed pitcher. The right-handed pitch is first accelerated by the posterior serape (right leg to left shoulder) during the windup and stride. The cocking and acceleration phases use the anterior serape muscles that diagonally cross from the left leg to the right shoulder: the left hip flexors and adductors, left internal oblique, right

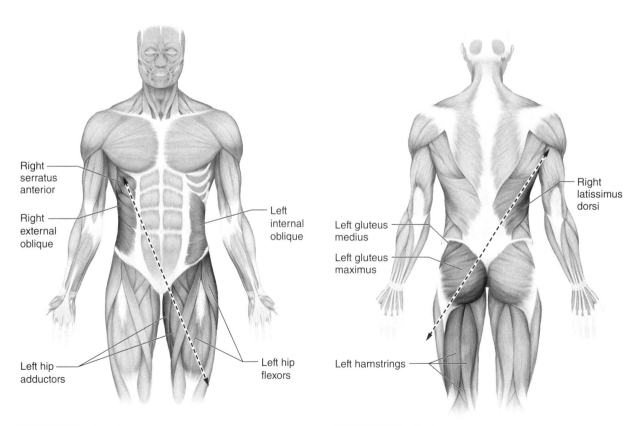

Right serratus anterior

Right external oblique

Left internal oblique

Left hip adductors

Left hip flexors

Left gluteus medius

Left gluteus maximus

Right latissimus dorsi

Left hamstrings

FIGURE 2.9   Anterior serape.

FIGURE 2.10   Posterior serape.

external oblique, and right serratus anterior. The right-handed pitch is decelerated by the posterior serape muscles that diagonally cross from the left leg to the right shoulder: the left soleus, left gastrocnemius, left hamstrings, left glutes, and right latissimus dorsi.

This diagonal acceleration and deceleration is an orchestrated event that is found in all sports, especially when rotation is used. For example, the same musculature that decelerates a right-handed pitch can accelerate a right-handed backhand in tennis.

Once you understand the diagonal nature of the anterior and posterior serape, you start to realize how all sport movements, as well as the four pillars, get their power. With this understanding, functional training for sport becomes as simple as training the power highways of the serape. Let's look at a training system designed to train the power highways.

JC's Training Octagon

Learning the inner workings of the serape can take a little time, and learning how to train it can take even more time. I developed my training octagon to make training the serapes easy.

If you combine the four pillars of human movement, the bow analogy, and the anterior and posterior serape models, you realize the body bends and rotates in eight directions and thus can perform practically any sport skill. These eight directions are the power highways. As you can see in figure 2.11, lines 1, 2, and 8 point to the direction of movement that predominantly uses the back musculature to extend the body. Lines 4, 5, and 6 predominately use front muscles to flex the body. Lines 3 and 7 use combinations of front and back muscles to cause a net horizontal rotation. When we say *predominantly*, we don't mean *exclusively*; all of these systems are integrated and help each other. We have oversimplified this model to make it easy to understand.

Table 2.7 brings everything together, including the eight power highways of the octagon, the main muscle systems involved in the movement, the sport skills associated with the movement, and some exercises that can improve the movement.

As you can see, the training octagon offers a simple biomechanical model and training system that any strength coach or athlete can use to train functionally. For example, by simply going to the sport skills column and selecting a movement you need to train, you can find a suitable exercise in the exercises column. Other columns provide additional information, such as muscle system used and direction of movement.

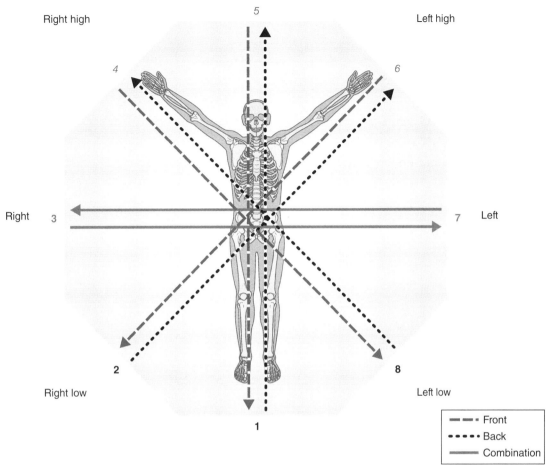

Right high

5

Left high

4

6

Right   3

Left   7

2

8

Right low

1

Left low

- - - Front
··· Back
— Combination

FIGURE 2.11 JC's training octagon.

TABLE 2.7 JC's Training Octagon

Number	Direction of movement	Muscles involved	Sport skills	Exercises
1	Low to high	Hamstrings, glutes, paraspinal muscles	Vertical and long two-leg jumps, lifting (ground up)	Squat, MB wood chop, good morning, deadlift, lunge, SB hyperextension, SB reverse hyperextension, SB bridge, KB swing, superman
2	Low right to high left	Right hamstrings, right glutes, left latissimus dorsi	Left backhand, right forehand, right-leg plant to cut left, decelerating left-hand throw	Left-hand cross low row, right-leg reaching lunge, right-leg CLA anterior reach, BP low-right-to-high-left chop, MB low-right-to-high-left chop, BP right-leg staggered-stance left-arm row

> continued

TABLE 2.7 > *continued*

Number	Direction of movement	Muscles involved	Sport skills	Exercises
3	Right to left (combined low right to high left and high right to low left)	Same as 2 and 4	Right-hand batting swing, right-leg-plant running, decelerating left-hand batting swing	BP short right-to-left rotation, MB right-to-left rotational throw, left-side SB skier
4	High right to low left	Right serratus anterior, right external oblique, left internal oblique, left hip flexors and adductor complex	Right-hand throw or serve, left-leg kick	High-right-to-low-left cable chop, right-arm-to-left-leg cross crunch or V-up, left-leg cross knee tuck, BP staggered-stance right-arm press
5	High to low	Bilateral hip flexors, abs	Pike or knee tuck in diving or gymnastics, guard work in grappling	Sit-up, crunch, V-up, knee tuck, SB and MB ball exchange
6	High left to low right	Left serratus anterior, left external oblique, right internal oblique, right hip flexors and adductor complex	Left-hand throwing or serving, right-leg kicking	High-left-to-low-right cable chop, left-arm-to-right-leg cross crunch or V-up, right-leg cross knee tuck, BP staggered-stance left-arm press
7	Left to right (combined low left to high right and high left to low right)	Same as 6 and 8	Left-hand batting swing, left-leg-plant running, decelerating right-hand batting swing	BP left-to-right short rotation, MB left-to-right rotational throw, right SB skier
8	Low left to high right	Left hamstrings, left glutes, right latissimus dorsi	Right-hand backhand, left forehand, left-leg plant to cut right, deceleration of right-handed throw	Right-hand cross low row, left-leg CLA anterior reach, left-leg reaching lunge, BP low-left-to-high-right chop, MB low-left-to-high-right chop, staggered-stance right-arm row

Conclusion

This chapter has laid the framework for how functional training can enhance sport performance. From basic definitions to the biomechanical discussion of the four pillars and the training octagon, the information allows the athlete and coach to better understand functional training and how to evaluate and design exercises and programs. Collectively, the information in these first two chapters sets the stage for the exercises and programs outlined in the rest of the book.

CHAPTER 3

The Performance Continuum

People often ask, "When can I start functional training?" My answer to that question has always been, "Yesterday!" I have been invited to speak on several professional panels regarding functional training, and over time I have come across professionals who believe that functional training should be placed within some sequence of training. Others suggest that functional training is an advanced method that one should attempt only after completing a general training phase using machine resistance. Still others argue that functional training is effective only during the rehabilitation phase and that traditional training methods such as Olympic lifting and powerlifting should be the staples of strength training. Some even think that functional training is sport-specific training that should be used sparingly during the off-season and preseason. Although these opinions can work their way into training methods and produce some success, the question remains: What is the optimal way to use functional training?

Let's agree that successful athletes do all sorts of things to achieve their success, and maybe some even do minimal strength and conditioning. Let's also agree that we can find champions throughout history who didn't do much strength and conditioning training. Does that mean we shouldn't recommend well-programmed strength and conditioning (functional or not) to athletes? Although some greats of the past and even a few in the present may have relied on pure talent to dominate their sport, most professionals now agree that a strength and conditioning program is essential to athletic success.

As to what kind of strength and conditioning program is best, we can say for sure that the appropriate use of *all* training methods has always been the best approach to developing an optimal program—and that includes functional training. Therefore, functional training must be considered within a training philosophy, within a training system, and as a training method—but not at the exclusion of other training systems. This will always be our position on strength and conditioning.

Criteria for Functional and Effective Training

Coaches and trainers often wonder if an exercise is the right exercise or even an appropriate exercise for their athlete. Believe it or not, this is actually an easy question to answer. If an exercise has biomechanical specificity, can be performed without pain, can be performed with good form, and improves quality of movement from week to week, it is a functional and effective exercise!

Biomechanical Specificity

In previous chapters, we discussed the meaning of functional movement and the principle of specificity. We know that the more closely an exercise simulates the target activity, the more specific and functional it is. However, there are many effective exercises that do not fit this general principle. For example, the single-leg press and the SB single-leg bridge are two functional progressions that improve running speed without looking anything like running. These progressions work because specificity applies to a fraction of a movement just as much as it applies to the total movement. In the case of the SB single-leg bridge, the vertical loading of the running motion is obviously missing. However, this exercise still teaches the hamstrings to pull and extend the hip while simultaneously controlling flexion and extension. The fact that the SB single-leg bridge can be used by a runner who can't run due to shin splints or lower-back injury makes it one of the most powerful functional exercise progressions for running even though it looks nothing like running.

Pain-Free Training

Training without pain is paramount in strength and conditioning. Everyone appreciates mental toughness and working through pain during special competitive moments; however, training should remain pain free. Pain is one of the mechanisms the body uses to protect itself while repairing some structure or tissue. It limits the range of motion or the loading of a structure or tissue by altering movement patterns. Therefore, training through pain is training with an altered movement pattern. Teaching and reinforcing incorrect movement patterns can rob athletes of top performance and predispose them to further and possibly permanent injury. This is why we say to work around pain, not through it. The take-home message is this: Train pain free!

Good Control

Good control of correct movement is the reason why proper progression is a *must-have* and not a *nice-to-have*. Correct movement is essential for a multitude of reasons. From a performance perspective, it provides synergistic force production between muscles and muscle systems that translates into more strength and power. When muscles work in a more coordinated fashion, the body can produce more force with less effort. Correct movement also provides better distribution of force over more muscle systems. This means that no one joint or structure takes excessive loading, saving a significant amount of wear and tear in specific areas such as the knees. Good movement quality can also help prevent injury, greatly reducing the likelihood of noncontact injuries such as anterior cruciate ligament (ACL) tears.

Steady Progress

Traditionally, progress has been viewed as the amount of weight an athlete can lift. However, progress comes in many forms. Less pain, faster movement, heavier loads, and greater coordination are all forms of progress. When we look at training from a functional perspective, progress is less objectively quantified and more subjectively evaluated. It is hard to put down on paper how stability has improved in a single-leg anterior reach, how the body has improved its stiffness through the rotational transition of the T push-up, or how the rhythm of the pelvis and spine have improved in a reaching lunge. Yet all of these are examples of progress and are the improvements that lead to athletic enhancement.

The keys to progress are patience and progression. Most athletes and coaches agree on this, but few practice what they preach. The biggest mistake made in functional training, and dare I say in training in general, is a lack of progression, which is often due to a lack of patience. Trainers, coaches, and even athletes always want to move ahead to the more advanced exercise or the higher load. But the poor control associated with advancing too fast actually slows progress by preventing the athlete from getting enough volume of quality work. For example, everyone wants to do single-leg anterior reaches without spending enough time on staggered-stance anterior reaches. You get more work out of 20 good staggered-stance anterior reaches than you get out of 10 bad single-leg reaches. Therefore, to achieve steady progress, you are better off with a greater volume of the basic exercise if the quality is better.

Manipulating Functional Intensity

Knowing how to progress and regress an exercise allows us to match the perfect exercise intensity to an athlete's ability. You can use a few simple techniques to regress or progress the intensity of any exercise to match ability. These techniques use the operational environment previously discussed in this book, as well as the mechanical laws of physics, to add or reduce training load and intensity. Let's look at some of these practical tweaks that can make any exercise just right.

Manipulate the Speed of Movement

Altering the speed of movement can change the intensity of any exercise. Generally speaking, the faster an exercise is, the harder it is. This is because additional power is required to increase and then reduce the momentum produced by speed. This is especially true of power movements, such as jumps. A bodyweight jump requires more force during the takeoff and landing than a bodyweight squat does.

However, speed can work in another way during some strength exercises. Slowing the speed of an exercise can increase the time under tension and the work done, thereby increasing the intensity. For example, if an athlete can perform 10 pull-ups quickly, slowing them to three counts up and three counts down will increase the work done and reduce the repetitions to 4 or 5.

Manipulate the Lever Arm

The lever arm of an exercise is the distance from a fixed point to where a force is applied (figure 3.1). The longer the lever arm, the higher the load and the harder the exercise.

The most common use of the lever arm as a modification in functional exercises can be seen in the push-up. A full push-up on the floor is harder than a push-up performed with the hands on a bench or performed from the knees instead of the feet (figure 3.2). This is because the push-up on the floor provides the longest lever arm from the feet (the fixed point) to the shoulders (the distal point). The same approach applies to progressions such as flys versus bench presses and lateral raises versus shoulder presses.

Manipulate the Base of Support

Manipulating the base of support of an exercise can dramatically alter intensity. Increasing the base of support provides greater stability and balance, reducing the load at the stabilizing points and difficulty of the movement. Reducing the base of support puts greater stress on the supporting structure. For example, performing alternating biceps curls on one leg requires more core and hip stability to maintain the 7-frame compared with performing the same exercise on two legs. Because of the need to balance, the dumbbell movement also slows down, giving the biceps more time under tension (i.e., better hypertrophy stimulus).

Reducing the base of support (going from a four-point position to a three-point position) also increases the load on other supporting structures, even those not necessarily in contact with the ground, as in a three-point push-up (figure 3.3). During a three-point push-up, greater loads are not only seen at the supporting arm but also at the core, which must avoid rotating and collapsing.

Hopefully this information on pedagogy and progression allows you to appreciate how important coaching is to the development and safety of an

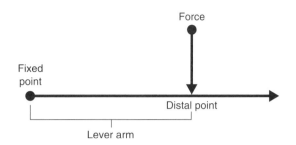

FIGURE 3.1 Lever arm.

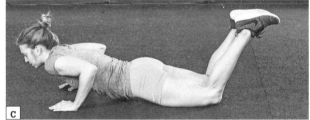
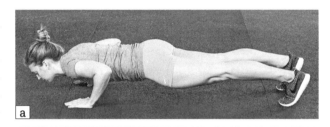
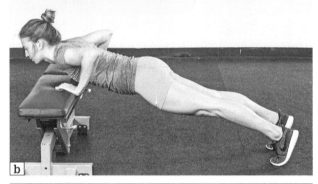

FIGURE 3.2 The push-up and lever arm: *(a)* full push-up on the floor; *(b)* push-up on a weight bench; *(c)* knee-modified push-up on the floor. Reducing the lever arm creates an easier progression of the push-up.

athlete. There is a reason why not just anyone can be a coach! It takes a lot of education, a systematic approach, patience, and discipline to provide the right instruction at the right time to facilitate the right execution for continual improvement in athletic performance. Because functional training is more instructionally intensive than other forms of strength training (such as machines and free weights), instruction, progression, and execution are particularly important.

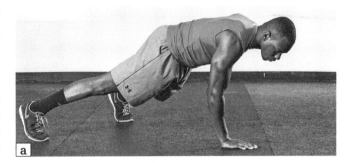

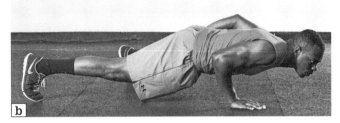

FIGURE 3.3 A three-point push-up places a higher demand on shoulder stability for the supporting arm and also develops excellent core stiffness.

Manipulate the Range of Motion

Adjusting the range of motion of an exercise can greatly alter its difficulty and training intensity. Larger ranges of motion, especially during slow and controlled movement where momentum does not play a significant role in producing movement, require more work and often greater control. An example of this can be seen in the reaching and single-leg squat progressions. A reach to the foot is harder than a reach to the knee, and a deep single-leg squat is harder than a partial single-leg squat. Just a few inches in depth or range can turn a novice exercise into an advanced exercise. This easy and immediate change in intensity makes this tweak effective in performing pyramid sets, where a few repetitions are done at the hardest intensity, a few are done at a medium intensity, and the rest are done at an easy intensity.

Being able to adjust a simple exercise from novice to advanced with just a few inches of movement is a powerful tool when working with athletes of varying levels. This tweak is a lifesaver during group training, as well as in the personal training world, where clients differ in abilities and sometime work in pairs and small groups.

Other Manipulation Strategies

There are other ways to regress or progress the intensity of functional exercises. The most obvious is adding external resistance such as a dumbbell, medicine ball, or band or pulley to increase the training intensity. Adding movement such as stepping and rotation to certain exercises (e.g., band presses, band rows) can also increase the intensity of the progression. Adding a stimulus such as a vibration platform or an oscillating bar can increase the difficulty of exercises such as squats and anterior reaches. Vibration can add instability and extra proprioception that enhance the communication between muscles and muscle systems. This improved communication can then be translated to function through specific functional exercises. However, vibration does not provide a free pass as functional training. It must be used for specific reasons and applications, some of which are beyond the scope of this text.

Other strategies for manipulating the intensity of functional training include moving in targeted and specific planes of motions or using specific drivers to facilitate desired movement patterns. For example, the single-leg anterior reach can be intensified by performing the reach to the front and to each side in what is called an *ABC pattern*. This pattern forces the hip into greater rotation as the athlete reaches to the outside and inside of the base foot.

Evaluation of Movement Patterns

Much has been made of movement assessments recently. Although some form of assessment is necessary to identify where athletes are in the functional spectrum, functional assessments have become overly complicated, offering athletes, coaches, and trainers little in the way of meaningful training information. Some movement evaluation systems have numbers associated with execution quality to provide a numeric score.

I have not yet found a movement evaluation that correctly predicts or assesses performance or injury susceptibility. Dr. Stu McGill, one of the world's leading authorities on spinal stability, has studied some of these assessments and found similar results. Additionally, many of these assessments use nonfunctional positions (e.g., overhead squat) and try to extrapolate functional information from these positions. In my opinion, using a test such as an overhead squat to assess the function of the body is equivalent to using a gymnast's iron cross on the rings to assess the function of the shoulder. Although some evaluation techniques within the available systems may be useful for gathering information pertinent to an exercise program, no system that I have looked at thus far has had everything I need. Therefore, I have created my own.

The movement system I use to evaluate an athlete's place on the movement spectrum is similar to an interview that is used to figure out if a person is right for a job. There is no number to assign, there are no specific predictors of performance or injury, and all movements have to be related to a specific function or the training for that function. In my assessment approach, the movement (i.e., assessment) is the training and the training is the movement. I don't care if the improvement comes from learning the movement or acquiring new strength that improves the movement; at times both of these factors become one and the same.

I have chosen eight basic exercises for assessing and training the four pillars of human movement and thus the Big Four sport movements. This way the training provides continuous assessment, and continuous assessment provides continuous training and thus continuous performance enhancement. Every set and repetition of these exercises is an opportunity to evaluate a pillar while also improving that pillar. For each of the eight progressions, I provide the purpose of the exercise, muscles worked, movement instructions, and cues from the important views of the movements (i.e., front, side, back). I also provide some common deviations seen in practice, their general causes, and exercises that address the deviations, strengthening whatever muscles may be weak. Finally, I provide a realistic goal that makes a great foundation from which to continue your functional training program.

The first exercise used to fix any deviation is the exercise that shows you the deviation. Simply use the manipulation strategies provided to regress the intensity of the exercise and remove the deviation, and repeat the exercise in its correct form. Eventually the body gets used to the correct form. As the movement quality improves, more strength is expressed, and progressions that were once impossible become easier to perform.

> **DISCLAIMER**
>
> This evaluation process is also a great coaching tool that can be used to evaluate and teach any other functional movement. However, it is not an orthopedic evaluation of muscular or orthopedic problems. If you have pain, discomfort, or any issue that does not allow the proper completion of any of these progressions, stop and contact an orthopedic specialist and a physical therapist for a complete biomechanical evaluation.

Single-Leg CLA Anterior Reach

The single-leg contralateral-arm (CLA) anterior reach is the most popular exercise to improve and assess locomotion. This exercise works single-leg hamstring, glute, and paraspinal coordination. It is particularly effective at teaching the hamstrings to extend the hip and control knee flexion and extension, as they do during the pulling phase of running. The single-leg position also provides the 7-frame hip stability so important to any locomotive skill.

Balance on your left leg and raise your right hand. Hinge at the hips and reach down as far as possible with good control (figure 3.4). Knee level can be used for beginners and shin level for intermediate athletes. Foot level will challenge just about anyone.

From the front, look for the 7-frame position made possible by a stable hip. Notice that the hip, knee, and foot are aligned and the hips are stable and parallel to the ground (i.e., creating a 7). From the side, look for a flat, stable foot and a slightly flexed knee aligned over the foot. Most of the movement should come from hinging the hip while keeping the knee slightly flexed. The back is straight

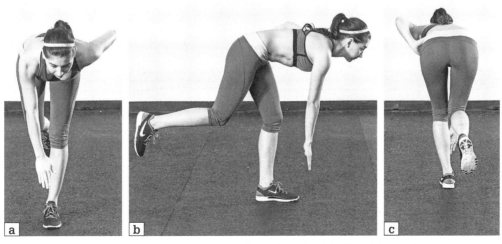

FIGURE 3.4 Single-leg CLA anterior reach: *(a)* front view; *(b)* side view; *(c)* rear view.

or slightly flexed so that the movement is always pain free. From behind, look for a parallel alignment of the shoulders and hips throughout the entire movement.

Major Faults

- Knees going in indicates weak hamstrings, glutes, and paraspinal muscles.
- Heels going up indicates weak calves, hamstrings, glutes, and paraspinal muscles.
- Hips posteriorly tilting (from side view) or shifting right or left (from rear view) indicates weak hamstrings, glutes, and paraspinal muscles.

Corrective Exercises

For weak glutes, hamstrings, and paraspinal muscles, perform the following:

- Single-leg squat
- All lunges (traditional and reaching variations)
- All deadlift and compound row variations using dumbbells, a barbell, or band or pulley
- SB bridge, SB hyperextension, and SB reverse hyperextension

For weak calves, perform the following:

- All marches
- 45-degree calf pump

Foundational Goal

For each leg, perform 10 repetitions in less than 15 seconds without the free leg touching the ground.

Loaded Single-Leg CLA Anterior Reach

This exercise can be loaded with dumbbells or a band or pulley to make it a perfect progression for strength development.

Single-Leg Squat

Similar to the single-leg CLA anterior reach, the single-leg squat is a fundamental exercise used to improve the 7-frame and all aspects of single-leg activities, especially when putting forces into the ground during the plant phase of running. Unlike the single-leg CLA anterior reach, the single-leg squat uses more knee flexion, which increases the focus on the quadriceps.

Balance on the right leg while holding the left leg back for counterbalance. The hands can remain on the hips or reach out to the front for counterbalancing. Flex equally from the ankle, knee, and hip and drop the knee of the free leg as low as it will go while maintaining control (figure 3.5).

From the front, look for the 7-frame made possible by a stable hip and good knee alignment. Notice that the hip, knee, and foot are aligned and the hips are stable and parallel to the ground (i.e., creating a 7). From the side, look for a flat, stable foot and equal contribution from ankle, knee, and hip flexion. The back stays straight throughout the movement and the movement is always pain free. From behind, look for a parallel alignment of the shoulders and hip throughout the entire movement.

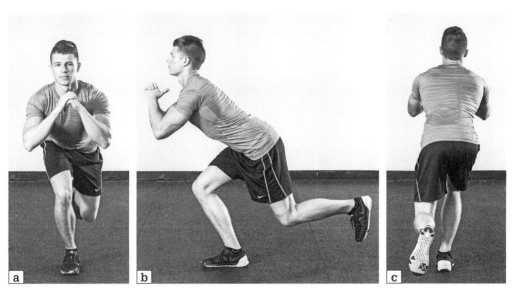

FIGURE 3.5 Single-leg squat: *(a)* front view; *(b)* side view; *(c)* rear view.

Major Faults

- Knees going in indicates weak hamstrings, glutes, and paraspinal muscles.
- Heels going up indicates weak calves, hamstrings, glutes, and paraspinal muscles.
- Hips posteriorly tilting (from side view) or shifting right or left (from rear view) indicates weak hamstrings, glutes, and paraspinal muscles.

Corrective Exercises

For weak glutes, hamstrings, and paraspinal muscles, perform the following:

- Single-leg CLA anterior reach
- All lunges (traditional and reaching variations)
- All deadlift and compound row variations using dumbbells, a barbell, or a band or pulley
- SB bridge, SB hyperextension, and SB reverse hyperextension

For weak calves, perform the following:

- All wall marches
- 45-degree calf pump

Foundational Goal

For each leg, perform 5 repetitions with the knee flexed 90 degrees or 1 full squat (rear knee touches the floor with the foot touching the floor).

Loaded Single-Leg Squat

This exercise can be loaded with dumbbells or a medicine ball to make it a perfect progression for strength development.

Bodyweight Double-Leg Squat

The squat is a fundamental exercise used to improve all aspects of level changes and lifting mechanics. It is excellent for developing the lower body and the posterior core musculature.

Place your feet slightly wider than shoulder-width apart. The hands can be behind the head, on the hips, or reaching out to the front for counterbalancing. Keeping the back straight, initiate the squat with a hip hinge, flexing equally from the ankle, knee, and hips (figure 3.6).

From the front, look for the A-frame made possible by the alignment of the shoulders, hips, knees, and feet. Notice that the hips, knees, and feet are aligned and the hips and shoulders are parallel to the ground. From the side, look for a flat, stable foot and equal contribution from ankle, knee, and hip flexion. The back stays straight throughout the movement. The movement is pain free. From behind, look for a parallel alignment of the shoulders and hips throughout the entire movement.

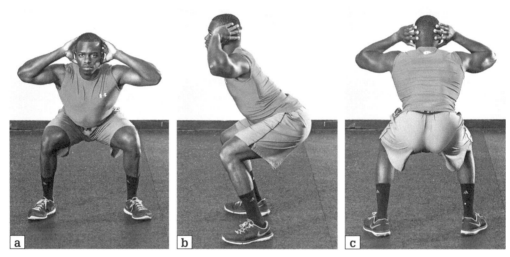

FIGURE 3.6 Bodyweight double-leg squat: (a) front view; (b) side view; (c) rear view.

Major Faults
- Knees going in indicates weak hamstrings, glutes, and paraspinal muscles.
- Heels going up indicates weak calves, hamstrings, glutes, and paraspinal muscles.
- Hips posteriorly tilting (from side view) or shifting right or left (from rear view) indicates weak hamstrings, glutes, and paraspinal muscles.

Corrective Exercises

For weak hamstrings, glutes, and paraspinal muscles, perform the following:
- Single-leg squat and single-leg CLA anterior reach
- All lunges (traditional and reaching variations)
- All deadlift and compound row variations using dumbbells, a barbell, or a band or pulley
- SB bridge, SB hyperextension, and SB reverse hyperextension
- MB ABC squat

For weak calves, perform the following:
- 45-degree wall march or run
- 45-degree calf pump

Foundational Goal

Perform 20 parallel squats in 20 seconds with no delayed onset muscle soreness (DOMS) the following day. A more athletic foundation, and one preferred for beginning athletes, is 3 sets of 20 squats with about 2 minutes rest between sets and with no DOMS the following day.

Loaded Double-Leg Squat

This exercise can be loaded with a barbell, dumbbells or kettlebells, or a medicine ball to make it a perfect progression for strength development.

Bodyweight Alternating Lunge

Due to its speed, alternating pattern, and greater eccentric component, the traditional alternating lunge is an intermediate progression for most people. For those who can't perform this progression, a split squat or a repeated single-side lunge could be a good starting point from which to progress to an alternating lunge. Not only does the traditional lunge strengthen the 7-frame and stretch the hip flexors of the trailing leg, it also requires the body to work on deceleration while changing levels.

From a standing position with feet together and parallel to each other, take a large step forward with one foot and bend both knees to lower the body toward the ground, ending in a split-squat position (figure 3.7). From there, push off the front foot and step back toward the rear foot to return to standing.

From the front, look for the A-frame alignment: perfect foot, knee, hip, and shoulder alignment with the hip and shoulder perfectly parallel to the ground. From a side view, the front shin should always remain vertical and the back knee should be aligned with or behind the hip and shoulder line. From the back, the

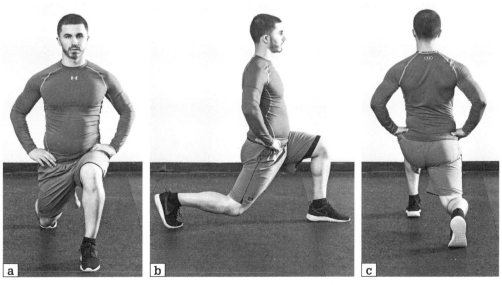

FIGURE 3.7 Bodyweight alternating lunge: *(a)* front view; *(b)* side view; *(c)* rear view.

shoulders should be parallel to the hips and the floor. Avoid any range of motion that creates pain in the knees or lower back.

Major Faults

- Front knee going in indicates weak glutes, hamstrings, and paraspinal muscles on that same side.
- Heel going up on the front foot indicates weak calves, glutes, hamstrings, and paraspinal muscles on that same side.
- Hips shifting right or left (from rear view) indicates weak glutes, hamstrings, and paraspinal muscles on the right or left side.

Corrective Exercises

For weak glutes, hamstrings, and paraspinal muscles, perform the following:
- All lunges
- All single-leg exercises
- All deadlift and compound row variations using dumbbells, a barbell, or a band or pulley
- SB bridge, SB hyperextension, and SB reverse hyperextension
- MB ABC squat

For weak calves, perform the following:
- 45-degree wall march or run
- 45-degree calf pump

Foundational Goal

Perform 20 alternating lunges (10 each leg) in 30 seconds without any DOMS the following day. A more athletic foundation, and one preferred for beginning athletes, is 3 sets of 20 alternating lunges with about 2 minutes rest between sets and without any DOMS the following day.

Loaded Alternating Lunge

This exercise can be loaded with a barbell, dumbbells or kettlebells, or a medicine ball to make it a perfect progression for strength development.

Bodyweight Push-Up

The bodyweight push-up is a fundamental pushing exercise in functional training. It's a great exercise for shoulder stability, upper-body strength, core stiffness, and lengthening of the hip flexors.

Start with hands on the floor under the shoulders, arms straight, and toes or balls of the feet on the ground. When ready, flex the elbows to lower the body to a level that maintains good technique (figure 3.8). Straighten the arms to return to the starting position.

From the front, see that the shoulders are parallel during the movement and there is no winging of the scapulae. From the side, see that the back is flat so the hips are in line with the shoulders and the low back is not sagging. If the back sags due to a weak front core, use a bench or other sturdy structure to elevate the hand support and shorten the lever arm, which reduces the amount of body

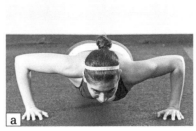
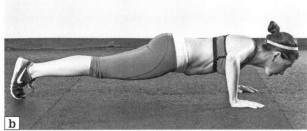
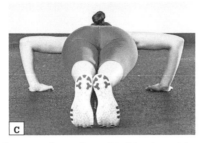

FIGURE 3.8 Bodyweight push-up: *(a)* front view; *(b)* side view; *(c)* rear view.

weight required to perform the push-up. Once the elevated bodyweight push-up is mastered with good technique and control, gradually lower the push-up to the ground. If there is pain in the wrists, shoulders, or elbows during the push-up, try elevating the hand support or using push-up grips for a pain-free exercise.

Major Faults

- Hips dropping (core collapse) indicates weak abs and hip flexors.
- Hips lifting indicates weak abs and hip flexors.
- Shoulder blades winging (shoulder blade collapse) indicates weak shoulder stabilizers during pushing.

Corrective Exercises

For weak abs and hip flexors, perform the following:
- All lunges
- All plank and push-up variations
- BP staggered-stance alternating press
- All knee-tuck variations
- V-up

For weak shoulder stabilizers during pushing, perform the following:
- All plank variations
- All push-up variations
- All BP pressing variations

Foundational Goal

Perform 15 to 20 perfect push-ups.

Instability Push-Up

This exercise can be made more difficult by performing it on an unstable surface such as a stability ball or two medicine balls or by going to a single-arm push-up.

Recline Pull (Row)

The recline pull focuses on the upper-back muscles and posterior core stability. It strengthens the pulling stability of the shoulders while developing core stiffness in the entire posterior core musculature. It also does a great job at developing grip strength as well as biceps strength.

Hold a bar or suspension equipment, such as an SBT System or ropes. Lie back so the body is in a straight line from shoulders to ankles. While retracting the shoulder blades and pushing the hips upward, pull up, bringing the chest toward the hands (figure 3.9). Control the movement down as the arms begin to straighten. Keep the shoulders retracted throughout the entire movement.

The resistance varies depending on the body position. The more upright the body is before the pull, the easier the exercise will be. As the body is lowered toward the ground, there will a noticeable increase in the resistance.

From the front, you should see a straight alignment of the body and symmetrical arm placement. From the side, the body should be straight. The hips should not drop when the bottom position is reached. From the back, the shoulder blades should be pulled back and should stay in place during the entire movement.

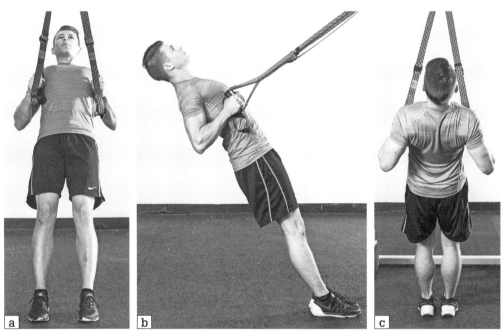

FIGURE 3.9   Recline pull (row): *(a)* front view; *(b)* side view; *(c)* rear view.

Major Faults

- Hips dropping at the bottom of the movement (core collapse) indicates weak hamstrings, glutes, and paraspinal muscles.
- Shoulder blades separating (shoulder blade collapse) indicates weak shoulder stabilizers during pulling.

Corrective Exercises

For weak glutes, hamstrings, and paraspinal muscles, perform the following:

- BP compound row
- SB bridge

- SB hyperextension and SB reverse hyperextension
- 45-degree back extension
- BP deadlift

For weak shoulder stabilizers during pulling, perform the following:

- All BP rows
- All dumbbell and kettlebell rows
- BP swim

Foundational Goal

Perform 15 to 20 perfect recline pulls (rows) at a 45-degree body angle.

Advanced Recline Pull (Row)

This exercise can be made more difficult by performing it using various handles and by going to a single-arm pull.

Rotation With Pivot

Rotation with pivot is one of the fundamental exercises used to develop hip rotation, also part of the fourth pillar. This exercise can be used to assess and strengthen hip mobility, specifically internal rotation. It is also a good exercise to include in a warm-up. The pivot motion can be added to many exercises, such as DB alternating shoulder presses or DB alternating curls, to add a hip-rotation component.

Start with your feet shoulder-width apart, arms in front of you with palms facing each other. Turn to the right so the hands go to the right side while pivoting the left foot to the right (figure 3.10). Return to the center, and then do the same to the left side.

From the front, the toes and knee of the stationary foot should point forward during the pivot. If the knee of the stationary leg turns out, limit the pivot to a range of motion where the knee and foot of the stationary leg stay pointing forward.

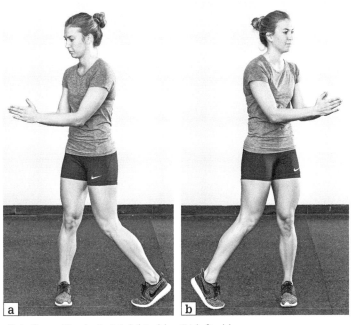

FIGURE 3.10 Rotation with pivot: *(a)* right side; *(b)* left side.

Major Faults

- A lack of coordination during the weight shift from right to left indicates a lack of body coordination.
- If the toes and knee of the stationary leg (the nonpivoting leg) point out, it indicates weak glutes in the rotational plane on the nonpivoting side.

Corrective Exercises

For lack of body control during the pivot, do the following:

- Perform all pivots to one side first and then to the other side.
- Do not perform alternating pivots.

For weak glutes in the rotational plane, perform the following:

- BP low-to-high chop
- DB or KB lateral reaching lunge
- MB short diagonal chop
- DB or KB cross overhead press with pivot

Foundational Goal

Perform 20 correct alternating repetitions (10 per side) without the knee or ankle on the stationary leg rotating out. In other words, internally rotate the hip without rotating the knee or ankle on the same side (i.e., pure internal hip rotation).

Loaded Rotation With Pivot

This exercise can be made more difficult by performing it against the resistance of a band or pulley or by holding a weighted implement such as a weight plate or medicine ball.

Rotation Without Pivot

Rotation without pivot is one of the fundamental functional exercises that develops core stiffness and the ability for the core to transfer forces between the hips and shoulders. You can use it to assess and strengthen the core stiffness necessary to transfer force from the hips to the shoulders, especially during rotational activities.

Hold your hands out in front of you with palms touching each other and arms extended. Starting from the ground up, your feet are hip-width apart, toes are forward, hips are locked in place, core is tight, arms are straight, and shoulders are facing forward. Imagine you are standing in the center of a clock, with 12 straight ahead. Move your hands left to 10 o'clock (figure 3.11) and then right to 2 o'clock without moving the feet or the hips. Keep the motion quick and smooth.

From the front, make sure the feet and hips aren't rotating with the hands and shoulders.

Major Faults

If the hips shake and move with the shoulders while the arms are moving, it indicates a lack of core stiffness.

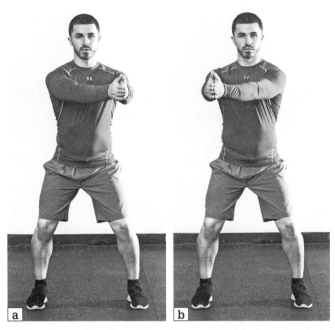

FIGURE 3.11 Rotation without pivot: *(a)* 10 o'clock; *(b)* 2 o'clock.

Corrective Exercises

For lack of core stiffness, perform the following:
- All planks
- All push-up variations
- All BP chops and short rotation variations
- All BP presses and rows

Foundational Goals

- Perform this exercise with good speed for 20 seconds without allowing the hips to shake.
- Perform any short 10-to-2-o'clock rotation without allowing the hips to shake.

Loaded Rotations Without a Pivot

This exercise can be made more difficult by performing it against the resistance of a band or pulley or by holding a weighted implement such as a weight plate or medicine ball.

Conclusion

This chapter has laid the foundation for learning and performing the appropriate functional training progression. Correctly executing the basic progressions that support the four pillars will result in an excellent evaluative tool, as well as set the stage for the proper execution of the exercises in this book. The upcoming chapters provide a wide selection of functional training exercises that expand on the basic eight progressions covered here.

PART II

Exercises

CHAPTER 4

The Essentials

We have now come to the anticipated part of the book—the training exercises. This chapter covers the top three functional training modalities: body weight, bands and pulleys, and dumbbells and kettlebells. For each modality, I provide the most common and effective exercises and the functional training best practices. Each exercise includes photos to illustrate the movement, details about the exercise, and instructions to support proper execution.

In the previous chapter, we discussed eight bodyweight exercises (i.e., the basic eight) that are used in the evaluation and training of the four pillars. The basic eight are also the primary progressions from which all other exercises in this book spring. It is essential to master the basic eight in order to easily learn and effectively perform the other exercises in this book.

The most important rule when performing the exercises in this book is to insist on no-pain training. Pain is our best ally in keeping us safe; stay away from pressure, discomfort, or pain and you will avoid problems. The next rule to follow is to initially execute all exercises with controlled, deliberate form. Once you master an exercise, perform the more dynamic or difficult versions. The biggest mistake in training is not mastering a movement before moving on to a more advanced progression. Take your time and focus on correct execution; the load and speed will naturally follow.

Body Weight

Before adding speed or loading the body externally, you need to ensure proper body position and control. This is why body weight is the most important modality to master. It is best to learn proper body mechanics first and then apply the good biomechanics learned with bodyweight training to all other modalities. In this section, you will recognize some natural progressions of the basic eight (see chapter 3), adding speed, increased range of motion, multiple planes of motion, and a reduced support base.

Step-Up

Details and Benefits

- This is a great basic progression to all single-leg work.
- Develops 7-frame hip stability and hip extension.
- Develops running speed and helps prevent hamstring injuries.
- Difficulty can be adjusted with step height; the higher the step, the harder the exercise.
- Start with a step height that allows you to step up without pushing off the rear leg.

Starting Position

- Stand on the floor with the step or box in front of you.
- Place your right foot flat on the step or box (figure 4.1a).

Movement

- Using only the right leg, step onto the step or box with your left leg (figure 4.1b).
- Using only the right leg, step down to the floor with the left leg.
- Do not use the left leg to push off the ground.
- Repeat the stepping action for the desired repetitions or time and perform on both sides.

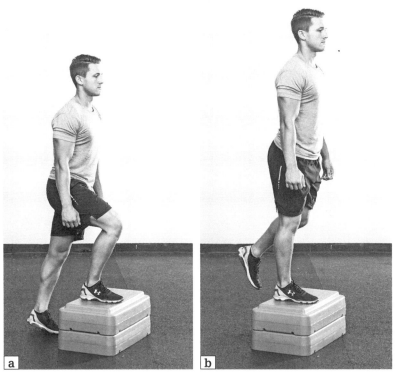

FIGURE 4.1 Step-up: *(a)* starting position; *(b)* step onto box or step.

Loaded Step-Up

This exercise can be loaded with dumbbells or a medicine ball.

Single-Leg Push-Off

The step-up can be performed explosively as the single-leg push-off. This is a great power developer and a complement to the split jump. Put your right foot on the step or box and perform an explosive step-up, powering through the extension until your entire body is airborne. Do not use the left leg to push off the ground. Land with the right foot on the box and bring the left foot back to the ground. Repeat the push-off with the right leg for the desired repetitions or time and perform on both sides.

Runner's Reach

Details and Benefits

- More advanced progression to the single-leg CLA anterior reach
- Develops 7-frame hip stability
- Great for developing running speed and preventing hamstring injuries

Starting Position

- Stand on your left leg with the left knee bent about 20 degrees, as if you were running.
- Allow the right leg to move back as the shoulders lean forward.
- Place your arms in a running position—right arm forward, left arm back—with elbows at 90 degrees (figure 4.2a).

Movement

- Extend the body while bringing the left arm forward and the right arm back.
- While the arms are moving, also bring the right knee forward and right foot up. Use a "knee up, toe up" cue to the top of the running position (figure 4.2b).
- At the top of the movement, you should be on the ball of the left foot with the left knee fully extended (figure 4.2c). The right knee is up, the right toe is up, the left arm is forward, and the right arm is back with both elbows at 90 degrees.
- Return to the starting position and repeat.

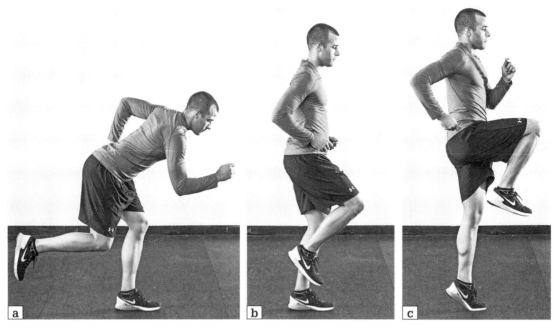

FIGURE 4.2 Runner's reach: *(a)* starting position; *(b)* middle position; *(c)* top of movement.

Single-Leg Rotational Squat

Details and Benefits
- More advanced multiplanar progression of the single-leg squat in chapter 3
- Great for developing single-leg rotational control to help prevent ACL injuries

Starting Position
- Stand on your left leg with the left knee slightly bent.
- Bring the right leg up so the thigh is parallel to the ground and the foot is pointing up (figure 4.3*a*).
- Hold your arms in any comfortable position that helps maintain balance (e.g., on hips).

Movement
- Keeping the left knee facing forward, squat on the left leg as you rotate the right knee to the right until it points to the right side of your body (figure 4.3*b*).
- Externally rotate the left hip as you turn so your left knee stays pointing forward.
- Perform on both sides of body.

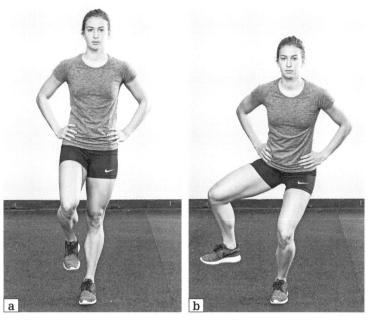

FIGURE 4.3 Single-leg rotational squat: *(a)* starting position; *(b)* squat and rotate right knee.

Plank

Details and Benefits
- Prerequisite to the push-up
- Great for core stiffness and shoulder stability

Starting Position
- Assume a stabilized push-up position, balancing between the hands and the balls of the feet (figure 4.4).
- You may perform this exercise on a soft surface from the elbows or use push-up handles if you have any wrist issues.

Movement
- Hold the position for the time prescribed.
- Make sure the lower back does not hyperextend.
- Make sure the shoulder blades are flat and not winging.

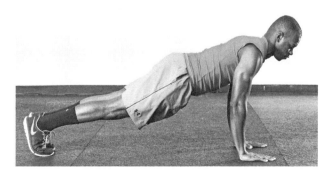

FIGURE 4.4 Plank.

Side T Plank

Details and Benefits

- Prerequisite to all push-ups
- Great for core stiffness and shoulder stability

Starting Position

- Assume a stabilized push-up position, balancing between the hands and balls of feet.
- Rotate to the left, balancing on the right hand, while keeping the inside of the left foot and the outside of the right foot flat on the ground. Point the left arm up to the ceiling, forming a sideways T (figure 4.5).
- You may perform the exercise on a soft surface from your elbows or use push-up handles if you have wrist issues.

Movement

- Hold the position for the time prescribed.
- Make sure the core does not sag or collapse through the movement.
- Perform on both sides of the body.

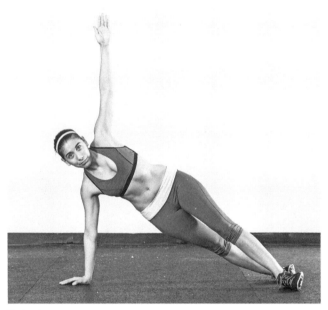

FIGURE 4.5 Side T plank.

Single-Arm Eccentrics

Details and Benefits

- Prerequisite to the single-arm and MB crossover push-ups
- Advanced progression for developing superior chest, shoulder, and core strength

Starting Position

- Assume a stabilized push-up position, balancing between the hands and the balls of the feet.
- Lift the left arm off the ground and balance on the right hand in a three-point plank (figure 4.6a).
- You may use push-up handles if you have wrist issues.

Movement

- Flex your left shoulder and elbow so as to slowly lower your body until your chest touches the ground (figure 4.6b). Slow the movement as much as possible.
- Use both arms to get back to a four-point plank position. Then balance on the left arm again and repeat the eccentric motion.
- Perform on both sides of body. For advanced training, you may perform all repetitions with the right arm before performing them with the left arm. For a lower intensity, alternate the repetitions, performing one with the right arm and then another with the left arm.

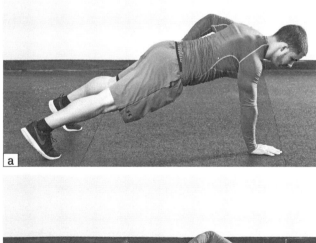

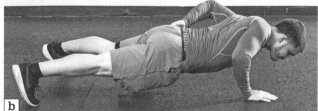

FIGURE 4.6 Single-arm eccentrics: *(a)* starting position in three-point plank; *(b)* lower the body.

T Push-Up

Details and Benefits

- More advanced progression of the push-up, combining the traditional push-up and side plank
- Develops shoulder stability and rotational core stiffness

Starting Position

- Assume a stabilized push-up position (figure 4.7a).
- Balance between the hands and the balls of the feet.

Movement

- Flex the elbows and lower the body until the chest is a few inches above the floor (figure 4.7b).
- Extend the arms and push up, simultaneously rotating to the right and balancing on the left hand, keeping the inside of the right foot and the outside of the left foot flat on the ground. Point the right arm up to the ceiling, forming a sideways T (figure 4.7c).
- Rotate back to the left and put the right hand on the floor. Perform a push-up, and then rotate to the left and balance on the right hand, keeping the inside of the left foot and the outside of the right foot flat on the ground. Point the left arm up to the ceiling, forming a sideways T. Continue to alternate sides.
- You may use push-up handles if you have wrist issues.

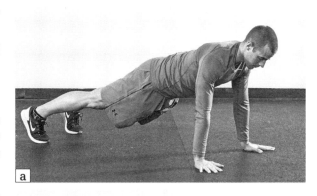

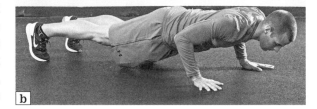

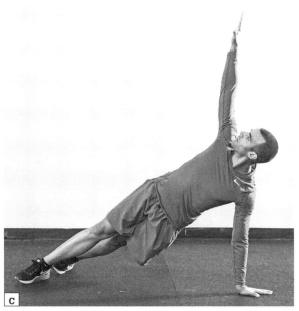

FIGURE 4.7 T push-up: *(a)* starting position; *(b)* lower the body; *(c)* push up and rotate.

Dip

Details and Benefits

- More advanced progression of push-ups and planks
- Develops shoulder stability and flexibility along with chest and triceps strength

Starting Position

- Stand on a box or other sturdy structure so that you are positioned between two parallel bars about shoulder-width apart.
- Place your hands on the bars and grip the bars securely.
- Jump up so your feet are off the box, your body is stabilized and balanced between the two bars, and your arms are fully extended (figure 4.8a).

Movement

- Keeping the core tight and with a slight lean forward, flex the elbows and shoulders until the chest is a few inches above the hands (figure 4.8b).
- At the bottom of the dip, extend the arms and press up until the arms are fully extended.
- Repeat the dip motion.

Weighted Dip

This exercise may be loaded with a weight belt that can hold weight plates or dumbbells.

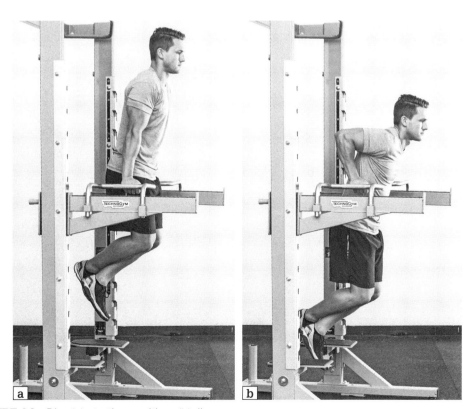

FIGURE 4.8 Dip: (a) starting position; (b) dip.

X-Up

Details and Benefits

- Dynamic progression from planks and push-ups
- Great complementary exercise to the BP high-to-low chop
- Develops the diagonal core musculature, making it excellent for kickers and combat athletes

Starting Position

- Lie flat on your back on the floor in an *X* position—arms and legs extended out to the sides with legs open and feet pointing out during the entire exercise.
- Brace the core before moving to stabilize the lower back.

Movement

- Simultaneously bring your right hand and left foot up so the right hand touches the arch of the left foot (figure 4.9*a*).
- Alternate right arm to left foot and left arm to right foot (figure 4.9*b*).
- The arms and legs should remain extended and the feet must face outward during the entire X-up motion.

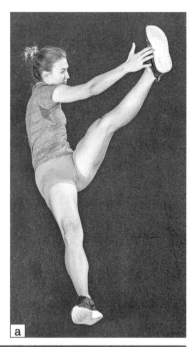

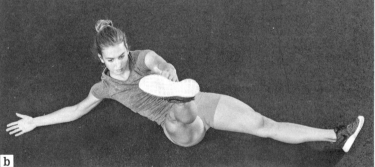

FIGURE 4.9 X-up: *(a)* right hand to left foot; *(b)* left hand to right foot.

V-Up

The V-up is a popular variation of the X-up, concentrating on more simultaneous, sagittal plane movement. Lie flat on your back, facing up and perfectly extended with hands overhead and feet together. Simultaneously flex your hips and bring your hands and feet together above your hip line, then back down to the extended position. Keep arms and legs fully extended throughout the exercise.

45-Degree Calf Pump

Details and Benefits

- Speed-specific version of the standard bodybuilding calf raise
- Excellent for developing the ankle stiffness needed for optimal running speed

Starting Position

- Stand in front of a wall.
- Put your hands on the wall with your arms extended. Assume a 45-degree lean and balance on the ball of the right foot.
- Bring the knee and foot up to the running position (figure 4.10a).

Movement

- Keeping the arms and core stiff and tight, perform mini ankle pumps without allowing the heel to come near the ground (figure 4.10b).
- Perform on both sides for time prescribed.

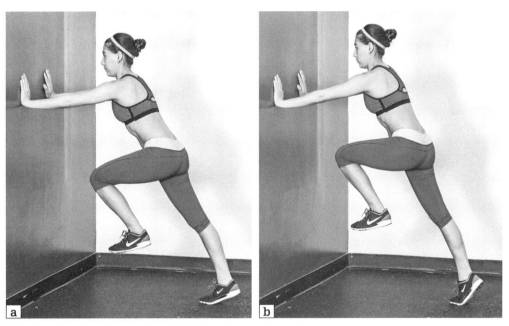

FIGURE 4.10   45-degree calf pump: *(a)* starting position; *(b)* ankle pump.

45-Degree Wall Run

Details and Benefits

- Natural progression to the 45-degree calf pump
- Excellent for developing locomotive core posture and ankle stiffness needed for acceleration power

Starting Position

- Stand in front of a wall.
- Put your hands on the wall with your arms extended. Assume a 45-degree lean and balance on the ball of the right foot.
- Bring the left knee and foot up to the running position (teaching cue: "Knee up, toe up") (figure 4.11a).

Movement

- Keep the arms extended and core stiff through the entire movement.
- Perform a fast running motion, simultaneously driving the left foot into the ground while bringing the right knee and foot up (teaching cue: "Knee up, toe up") (figure 4.11b).
- The feet must always land in the same spot so as not to lose body angle.
- Keep the ankles stiff, never allowing the heels to come near the ground.
- Continue the dynamic running motion for repetitions or time prescribed.

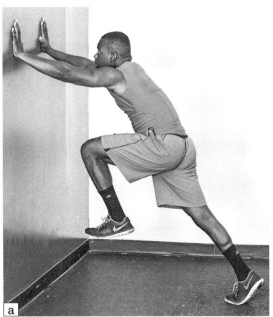 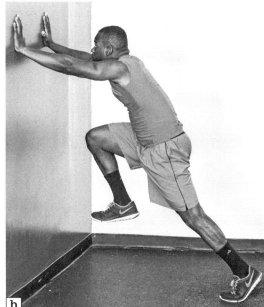

FIGURE 4.11 45-degree wall run: *(a)* starting position; *(b)* running motion.

Vertical Jump

Details and Benefits

- Natural progression from the bodyweight double-leg squat and complement to the MB reverse scoop throw
- Excellent for triple extension and the hip power needed for vertical jumps

Starting Position

- Stand up straight.
- Stand with your feet shoulder-width apart (feet may point slightly outward).
- The hands can remain behind the head (i.e., prisoner position), on the hips (figure 4.12a), or move freely at the sides to create a countermovement.

Movement

- Flex your knees and hips and squat down (figure 4.12b). Go as deep as needed for the counter loading movement. (Depth depends on the amount of elastic versus muscular strength you possess.) If you're using the arms for a countermovement, they come down and back at the bottom of the loading position.
- Explode up into a vertical jump, keeping the body fully extended while airborne (figure 4.12c). If you're using your arms to propel you, bring them overhead as you jump up.
- Land softly on both feet.

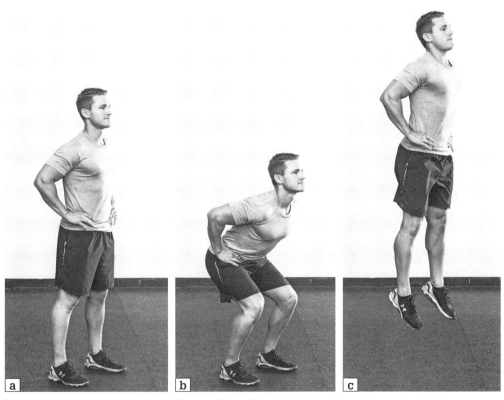

FIGURE 4.12 Vertical jump: *(a)* starting position; *(b)* squat; *(c)* jump.

Squat Jump

The squat jump is the vertical jump performed repeatedly without resting between jumps. It is effective for developing power endurance and increasing the metabolic demand on the lower body and cardiorespiratory system. To perform the squat jump, perform a vertical jump and land softly on your feet, but allow the downward momentum to immediately take you into the parallel squat position. When you're at the bottom of the squat, immediately jump again, and repeat for assigned number of repetitions.

Loaded Vertical Jump

This exercise can be loaded with dumbbells or medicine balls.

Alternating Split Jump

Details and Benefits

- Natural progression from bodyweight lunging progressions
- Excellent for hip strength and flexibility, making it a top deceleration exercise

Starting Position

- Stand up straight with hands behind the head (prisoner position), on your hips, or by the sides if you're going to use the arms for countermovement.
- The feet should be between hip- and shoulder-width apart and in a split stance (i.e., low lunge position) with the right foot forward (figure 4.13a).
- The split stance should be long enough to keep the right knee above the ankle and the left knee bent and behind the vertical shoulder–hip line. The left heel should be off the ground.

Movement

- Explode up into a vertical jump, simultaneously switching leg positions—left leg goes forward and right leg goes back (figure 4.13b). Keep the hands behind the head if maintaining the prisoner position. If using countermovement, move the arms as necessary to generate power and maintain balance.
- Land softly on both feet and allow the downward momentum to immediately take you into the split squat.
- Once you're at the bottom of the split squat, jump again.
- Repeat, alternating the split-jump motion.

Loaded Alternating Split Jump

This exercise can be loaded with a weighted vest, dumbbells, or medicine balls.

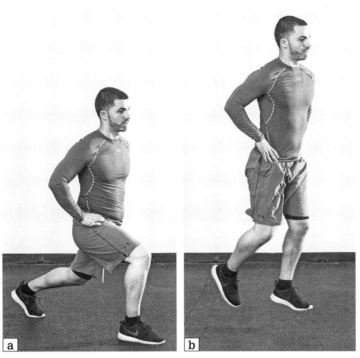

FIGURE 4.13 Split jump: *(a)* starting position; *(b)* vertical jump and leg switch.

Skater

Details and Benefits
- Natural progression to the DB or KB lateral reaching lunge in chapter 4
- Excellent for developing power for skating sports and for lateral changes of direction for field and court athletes, making it a top performer with skating and field athletes

Starting Position
- Stand on the right leg with the right knee and hip slightly bent.
- Lean forward at the shoulders with the left arm crossed in front of the body and the right arm back (figure 4.14a).

Movement
- Using your arms for counterbalance, jump to the left.
- Land on the left foot, stabilize your position with the right arm crossed in front of the body and the left arm back, and immediately jump back to the right (figure 4.14b).
- Repeat the lateral jumping motion, using your arms for counterbalance.

Weighted Skater
This exercise can be loaded with a weighted vest, dumbbells, or medicine balls.

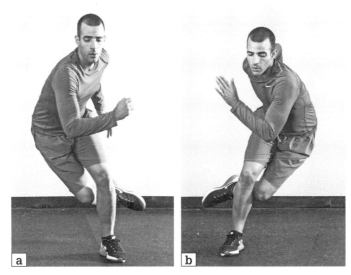

FIGURE 4.14 Skater: *(a)* jump to the left; *(b)* jump to the right.

Burpee

Details and Benefits

- Natural progression from the bodyweight double-leg squat and bodyweight push-up
- Excellent for strength and flexibility, making it a top performer as a level-change exercise for combat and field athletes

Starting Position

- Stand up tall with your arms at your sides.
- Keep the core tight throughout the movement.

Movement

- From a standing position, squat down and put your hands on the floor in front of you (figure 4.15a).
- Sprawl back into a plank position while keeping your core tight (figure 4.15b).
- Jump your feet back to their original position and stand up. Repeat.

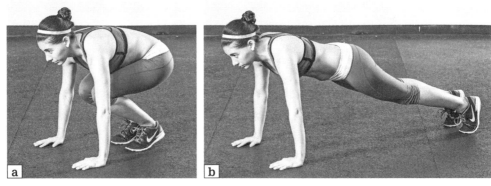

FIGURE 4.15 Burpee: *(a)* squat position; *(b)* push-up position.

Weighted Burpee

This exercise can be loaded with a weighted vest, dumbbells, or medicine balls. If using dumbbells, hold a dumbbell in each hand. During the squat, place the dumbbells on the ground under your hands as you jump back into plank. If using a medicine ball, hold the medicine ball in both hands and place it on the ground with both hands on the ball as you jump back to plank.

Explosive Push-Up

Details and Benefits

- Natural progression from the plank and bodyweight push-up
- Excellent for dynamic core stiffness and pushing power

Starting Position

- Assume a stable push-up position.
- Balance between the hands and the balls of the feet or toes.

Movement

- Flex the elbows and lower the body until the chest is a few inches above the floor (figure 4.16a).
- Explosively extend the arms and push off the ground, holding the arms extended throughout the time the body is off the ground (figure 4.16b).
- Land softly into a push-up position with the chest a few inches above the floor. Then explode back into the air.

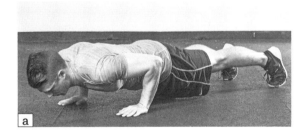

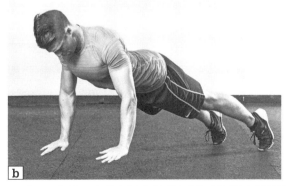

FIGURE 4.16 Explosive push-up: *(a)* Lower the body to the ground; *(b)* explosively extend the arms.

Bands and Pulleys

Once body weight is mastered, the next thing we do is control rotational movement and deceleration to the highest degree possible. To load the diagonal and horizontal vectors that control rotational movement, nothing beats bands and pulleys (BP). Pulleys, also called *cables*, offer constant mass and are preferred for the heavy, slow movements typically found in strength training. On the other hand, bands offer variable resistance and allow the explosive movements typically found in power training. Chapter 1 provides information on the best band products for functional training. Most of the exercises in this section can be done with either a band or a pulley.

Some nomenclature on positioning and movement will make it simpler to understand the following exercise descriptions. The name of the exercise is self-explanatory. As for descriptions, first I describe the base, then the total-body position (or movement), then the upper-body limb-holding pattern, and finally the movement itself. The reference position is standing upright, stable on two legs in a parallel position, with two hands holding a piece of equipment (e.g., band handles) and simultaneous upper-body movement. Anything beyond that position is described in the exercise name. For example, the name *BP deadlift* implies the exercise is based on two legs in a parallel stance and two hands are holding the handles. On the other hand, the BP staggered-stance CLA press implies the base is a staggered stance, the position is upright, and the press is performed by the arm opposite to the front foot (i.e., contralateral arm). Also, the loading point refers to where the load is coming from or where the band is attached. There are a few exceptions to this nomenclature, but the names will be obvious and descriptive of the exercise.

BP Deadlift

Details and Benefits

- Natural progression from the bodyweight double-leg squat, focusing on hip hinging
- Excellent hip-strengthening exercise with minimal knee involvement and reduced spinal compression
- Excellent for athletes with knee and certain back issues

Starting Position

- Set the loading point as close to the floor as possible.
- Facing the load, stand up tall with the handles in your hands and lean back to counterbalance the pull of the load (figure 4.17a).

Movement

- Keeping your back straight, sit back so your hips flex and slightly drop toward the ground as your shoulders move toward the loading point. Stop when you feel a comfortable pull on the hamstrings (figure 4.17b).
- While your hips are hinging, allow a slight flexion of the knees (10-15 degrees), keep the shoulder blades back, and allow the arms to reach and move the shoulders in the direction of the pull.
- Extend the hips and return to the starting position.

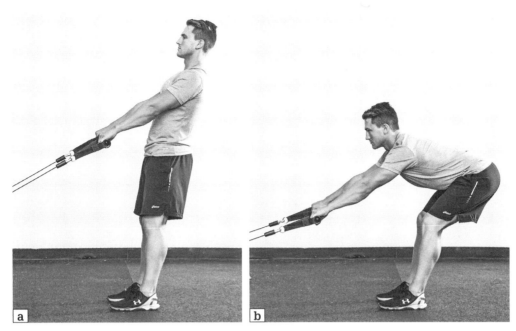

FIGURE 4.17 BP deadlift: *(a)* starting position; *(b)* sit back.

BP Staggered-Stance CLA Deadlift

Details and Benefits

- Natural progression from the single-leg CLA anterior reach and all reaching lunge progressions
- Great precursor to all staggered-stance rowing progressions
- Excellent unilateral back- and hip-strengthening exercise with minimal knee involvement and reduced spinal compression
- Popular with athletes who use low positions and low deceleration mechanics

Starting Position

- Set the loading point as low as possible and hold the handle in the left hand.
- Facing the loading point, stand up tall in a split stance, with the right leg forward and the knee over the ankle (figure 4.18a).
- The left leg is back, knee bent and behind the vertical shoulder–hip line, feet facing forward, and rear leg stable on the ball of the foot.

Movement

- Keeping your back straight, flex your hips and allow the arm and shoulder to move in the direction of the pull (figure 4.18b). Stop when you feel a comfortable pull on the right hamstring.
- Extend the hips and come back to the starting position.
- Make sure to keep both knees slightly flexed (10-15 degrees), keep the shoulder blades back, and maintain a tight core during the entire movement.
- Perform on both sides of the body.

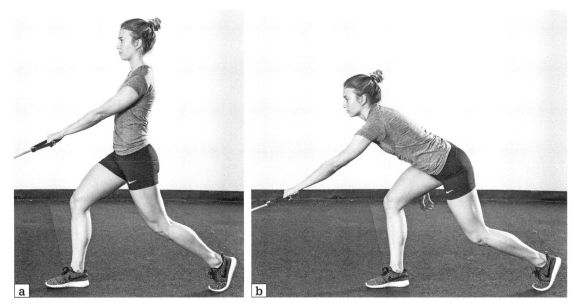

FIGURE 4.18   BP staggered-stance CLA deadlift: *(a)* starting position; *(b)* sit back.

BP Staggered-Stance CLA Press

Details and Benefits
- Natural progression from the bodyweight alternating lunge and bodyweight push-up
- Excellent anterior core and chest exercise
- Popular with runners and throwers

Starting Position
- Set the loading point about chest-height.
- Holding a handle in the right hand, turn away from the load and stand up tall in a split stance with both knees slightly flexed (10-15 degrees) and the left leg forward with the knee over the ankle.
- The right leg is back, knee bent and behind the vertical shoulder–hip line, feet facing forward, and rear leg stable on the ball of the foot.
- Keeping the core tight, hold the handle slightly outside the right side of the chest and right shoulder (figure 4.19a).

Movement
- Keeping the core tight, press the handle forward with the right hand without rubbing the band or cable on the outside of the upper arm (figure 4.19b).
- Repeat the pressing motion.
- Perform on both sides of the body, alternating leg positions.

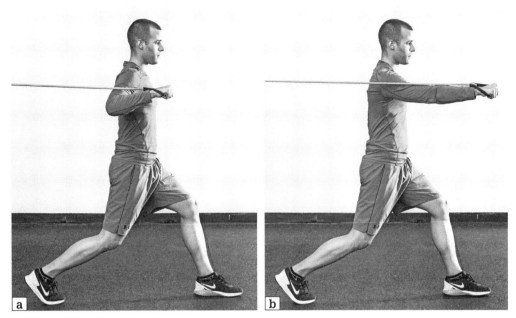

FIGURE 4.19 BP staggered-stance CLA press: *(a)* starting position; *(b)* press.

BP Staggered-Stance CLA Incline Press

The BP staggered-stance CLA incline press is great for runners and throwers to develop the anterior core and chest. The starting position and basic movement are the same as in the BP staggered-stance CLA press except the loading point is below the knees and you press the handle upward at a 45-degree angle (figure 4.20). Repeat and perform on both sides of the body, alternating leg positions.

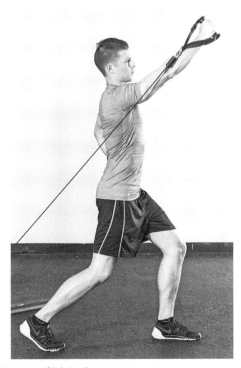

FIGURE 4.20 BP staggered-stance CLA incline press.

BP Staggered-Stance CLA Decline Press

Like the BP staggered-stance CLA press and the BP staggered-stance CLA incline press, the BP staggered-stance CLA decline press is perfect for runners, throwers, and combat athletes. The starting position and basic movement are the same as in the BP staggered-stance CLA press except the loading point is well above the head (figure 4.21a) and you press the handle downward at a 45-degree angle. Press the handle down at a 45-degree angle without rubbing the band or cable on the outside of the arm (figure 4.21b). Repeat and perform on both sides of the body, alternating leg positions.

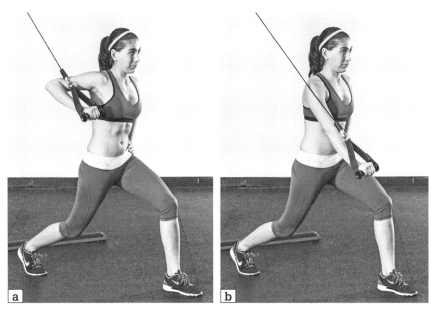

FIGURE 4.21   BP staggered-stance CLA decline press: *(a)* starting position; *(b)* press down.

BP Staggered-Stance Press

Details and Benefits
- Natural progression from the bodyweight alternating lunge and bodyweight push-up and a perfect complement to the previous staggered-stance CLA progressions
- Excellent anterior core and chest exercise
- Popular with runners and athletes in combative situations who need to push an opponent

Starting Position
- Set the loading point about chest-height.
- Holding a handle in each hand, turn away from the load and stand up tall in a split stance with both knees slightly flexed (10-15 degrees) and the left leg forward with the knee over the ankle.
- The right leg is back, knee bent and behind the vertical shoulder–hip line, feet facing forward, and rear leg stable on the ball of the foot.
- Keeping the core tight, hold a handle in each hand slightly outside of each chest and shoulder (figure 4.22a).

Movement

- Keeping the core tight, simultaneously press both handles forward without rubbing the band or cable on the outside of the upper arm (figure 4.22b).
- Repeat the pressing motion.
- Alternate leg positions and repeat.

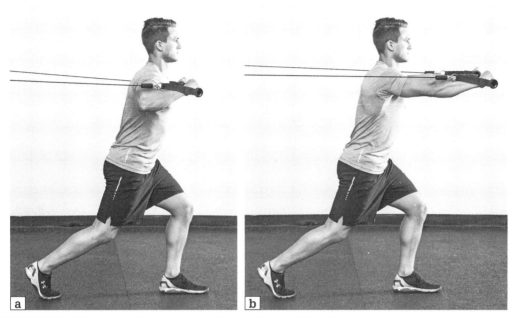

FIGURE 4.22 BP staggered-stance press: *(a)* starting position; *(b)* press.

BP Staggered-Stance Alternating Press

The BP staggered-stance alternating press shares the same benefits and features as the BP staggered-stance press, but the alternating pattern of the arms (figure 4.23) adds a rotational component. This exercise emphasizes the anterior serape musculature. After completing a set, switch leg positions and repeat.

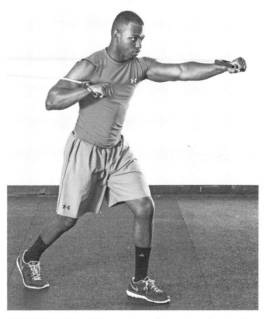

FIGURE 4.23 BP staggered-stance alternating press.

BP Staggered-Stance Fly

Details and Benefits

- Natural progression from the bodyweight alternating lunge, bodyweight push-up, and BP press
- Excellent prefatigue, anterior core, and chest exercise
- Popular with runners, throwers, and athletes in close, combative situations

Starting Position

- Set the loading point about chest-height.
- Hold a handle in each hand.
- Turn away from the load and stand tall in a split stance with both knees slightly flexed (10-15 degrees) and the left leg forward with the knee over the ankle.
- The right leg is back, knee bent and behind the vertical shoulder–hip line, feet facing forward, and rear leg stable on the ball of the foot.
- Keeping the core tight, hold the arms out to the sides with elbows slightly flexed, in line with the shoulders, and palms facing each other (figure 4.24a). Avoid over-stretching the chest and shoulders by not allowing the hands to reach behind the shoulder line.

Movement

- Keeping the core tight, arms out to the sides, elbows slightly flexed, and palms facing forward, bring the hands toward each other until they almost touch (figure 4.24b).
- The only movement should be at the shoulder joints.
- Brings the arms back to the outstretched position and repeat the fly motion.
- Perform with alternating leg positions.

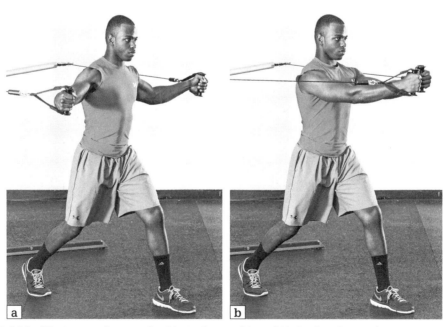

FIGURE 4.24 BP staggered-stance fly: (a) starting position; (b) bring hands together.

BP Row

Details and Benefits

- Most basic of all standing rowing motions
- Natural progression from the bodyweight double-leg squat and recline pull (row)
- Excellent fundamental exercise to work the entire backside of the body

Starting Position

- Set the loading point between chest- and knee-height. (The lower the loading point, the heavier the load can be.)
- Facing the loading point, stand tall in a parallel stance with feet shoulder-width apart.
- Hold a handle in each hand.
- Slightly flex the knees and lean back as necessary to counterbalance the load (figure 4.25a).

Movement

- Keeping your back straight and core tight, simultaneously pull the handles back until the hands are outside the chest (figure 4.25b).
- Return the hands to starting position.
- Repeat the rowing motion.

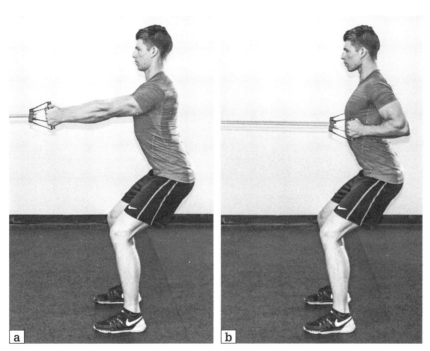

FIGURE 4.25 BP row: *(a)* starting position; *(b)* pull handles back.

BP Staggered-Stance Alternating Row

Details and Benefits

- Natural progression from and complement to anterior reaches, reaching lunges, and staggered-stance CLA rowing progressions
- Excellent core stiffness and hip exercise focusing on the rotational muscles of the core

Starting Position

- Set the loading point between chest- and hip-height.
- Facing the loading point, stand up tall and hold a handle in each hand.
- Stand upright in a split stance with both knees slightly flexed (10-15 degrees) and the left leg forward with the knee over the ankle.
- The right leg is back, knee bent and behind the vertical shoulder–hip line, feet facing forward, and rear leg stable on the ball of the foot.
- Pull the right handle until it is outside the right side of the chest while keeping the left arm straight (figure 4.26a).

Movement

- Simultaneously row with the left arm while extending the right arm (figure 4.26b).
- Repeat, alternating the rowing pattern.
- Switch legs and repeat.

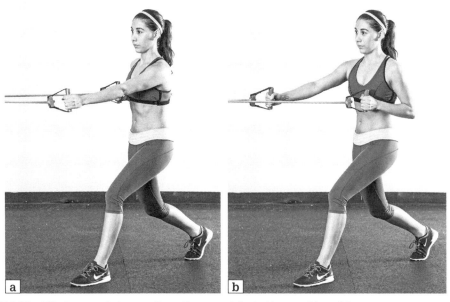

FIGURE 4.26 BP staggered-stance alternating row: (a) starting position; (b) row.

BP Staggered-Stance Bent-Over Alternating Row

Details and Benefits

- Natural progression from the bodyweight double-leg squat, recline pull, and BP deadlift
- Excellent hamstring, back, and shoulder strength and flexibility exercise
- Popular with swimmers, throwers, racket sport athletes, and grapplers

Starting Position

- Set the loading point between chest- and hip-height.
- Facing the loading point, stand up tall and hold a handle in each hand.
- Stand in a split stance with both knees slightly flexed (10-15 degrees) and the left leg forward with the knee over the ankle.
- The right leg is back, knee bent and behind the vertical shoulder–hip line, feet facing forward, and rear leg stable on the ball of the foot.
- Flex at the hips, keeping the back as straight as possible, feeling a good stretch in the left hamstring.
- Hold the arms overhead, pointing straight in the direction of the pull.

Movement

- Keeping the hips flexed and the left arm straight, pull the right handle until it's outside the right shoulder (figure 4.27a).
- Simultaneously extend the right arm and pull with the left (figure 4.27b).
- Keeping the hips flexed and back straight, repeat the alternating rowing motion.
- Perform with alternating foot positions.

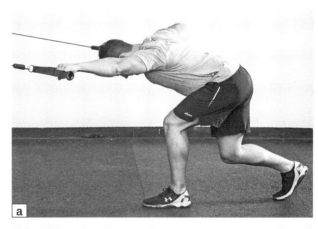

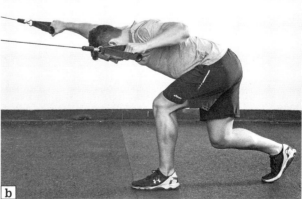

FIGURE 4.27 BP staggered-stance bent-over alternating row: (a) row with right arm; (b) row with left arm.

BP Compound Row

Details and Benefits

- Natural progression from the bodyweight double-leg squat; adds a focus on hip hinging and is a perfect transition from the BP deadlift
- Excellent hip- and back-strengthening exercise with minimal knee involvement or spinal compression
- Excellent for athletes who have knee and certain back issues

Starting Position

- Set the loading point as low as possible.
- Facing the load, stand up tall with handles in your hands.
- Lean back to counterbalance the pull of the load.

Movement

- Keeping your back straight, allow your hips to flex and move back as your shoulders come forward. Stop when you feel a comfortable pull on the hamstrings (figure 4.28a).
- While your hips are hinging, allow a slight flexion of the knees (10-15 degrees), keep the shoulder blades back, and allow both arms to reach in the direction of the pull.
- Extend the hips while simultaneously rowing with both arms until each hand is outside the chest (figure 4.28b).
- Repeat the compound rowing motion.

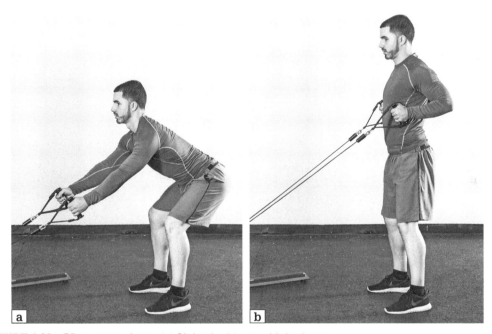

FIGURE 4.28 BP compound row: (a) Sit back; (b) row with both arms.

BP Staggered-Stance CLA Row

Details and Benefits

- Natural progression from the single-leg CLA anterior reach and DB or KB front reaching lunge later in this chapter
- Excellent back- and hip-strengthening exercise with minimal knee involvement
- Popular with athletes who use low positions, such as tennis players and wrestlers

Starting Position

- Set the loading point at hip-height and hold a handle in the left hand.
- Facing the loading point, stand up tall in a split stance with the right leg forward and the knee over the ankle, both knees slightly flexed (10-15 degrees) (figure 4.29a).
- The left leg is back, knee bent and behind the vertical shoulder–hip line, feet facing forward, and rear leg stable on the ball of the foot.

Movement

- Keeping your back straight, pull the left hand to the left side of the chest (figure 4.29b).
- Repeat the rowing motion.
- Perform on both sides of the body, switching foot positions.

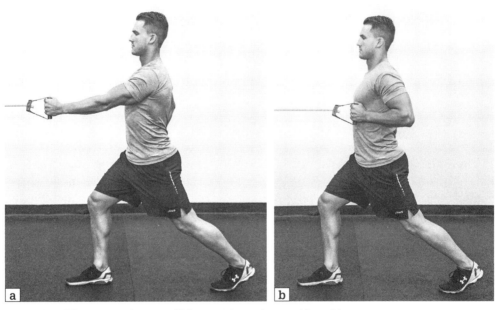

FIGURE 4.29 BP staggered-stance CLA row: *(a)* starting position; *(b)* row.

BP Staggered-Stance CLA High-to-Low Row

The BP staggered-stance CLA high-to-low row has the same benefits as the BP staggered-stance CLA row, but the setup and movement are slightly different. Set the loading point above your head and hold the handle in your left hand (figure 4.30a). Get into the starting split-stance position with the right leg forward. Keeping your back straight, pull the left hand down at a 45-degree angle until it reaches the left side of the chest (figure 4.30b). Repeat and perform on both sides of the body, switching foot positions.

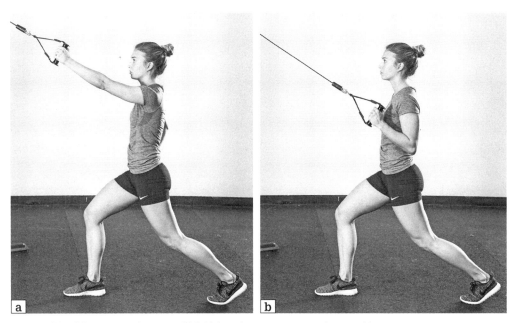

FIGURE 4.30   BP staggered-stance CLA high-to-low row: *(a)* starting position; *(b)* row.

BP Staggered-Stance CLA Low-to-High Row

The setup and movement for the BP staggered-stance CLA low-to-high row are slightly different than for the BP staggered-stance CLA row. Set the loading point as low as possible and hold the handle in your left hand. Get into the starting split-stance position with the right leg forward. Keeping your back and left arm straight, hinge at the hip and lean the shoulders forward until the core is perpendicular to the line of pull and you feel a good stretch in the left hamstring (figure 4.31a). Row with the left hand at a 45-degree angle until the left hand reaches the left side of the chest (figure 4.31b). Repeat the rowing motion to each side, switching foot positions.

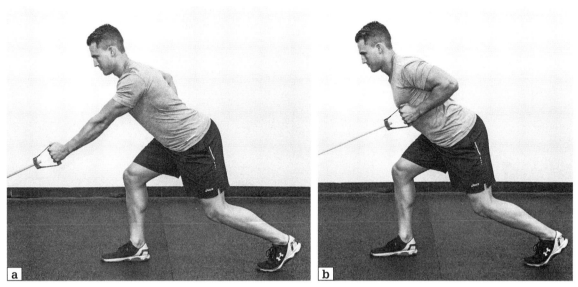

FIGURE 4.31 BP staggered-stance CLA low-to-high row: *(a)* starting position with hip hinge and lean; *(b)* row.

BP Staggered-Stance CLA Compound Row

The BP staggered-stance CLA compound row provides a double dose of unilateral glute training. It's a combination of the BP staggered-stance CLA row and the BP staggered-stance CLA deadlift, and the setup and starting position are the same as both. Get into the starting split-stance position with the right leg forward. Hold the handle in the left hand. Keeping your back and left arm straight, hinge at the hip and lean the shoulders forward until the core is perpendicular to the line of pull and you feel a good stretch in the right hamstring (figure 4.32a). While your hips are hinging, allow a slight flexion of the knees (10-15 degrees), keep the shoulder blades back, and allow the right arm to reach in the direction of the pull. Extend the hips while pulling the left hand to the left side of the chest (figure 4.32b). Repeat the compound rowing motion and perform on both sides of the body, switching foot positions.

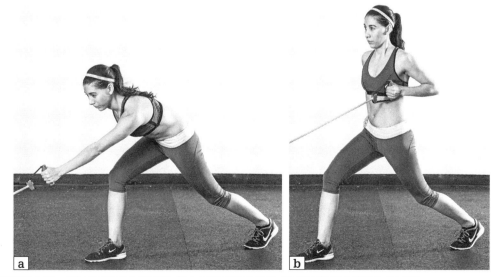

FIGURE 4.32 BP staggered-stance CLA compound row: *(a)* starting position; *(b)* row.

BP Swim

Details and Benefits

- Natural progression from the bodyweight double-leg squat, BP deadlift, and BP compound and bent-over progressions
- Excellent fundamental exercise to work the strength of the anterior core musculature and the flexibility of the posterior core musculature

Starting Position

- Set the loading point as high as possible, well above the head.
- Facing the loading point, stand up tall with the knees slightly bent and in a parallel stance, feet shoulder-width apart (figure 4.33a).
- Hold a handle in each hand with palms facing down.
- Keep your arms straight and pointing toward the loading point.

Movement

- Explosively flex the entire body into a crunch position.
- Keeping your arms straight, simultaneously pull your hands down and back (i.e., swim motion) until they are next to the hips and the bands or cables slightly touch the shoulders (figure 4.33b).
- Extend the body to the starting position and repeat.

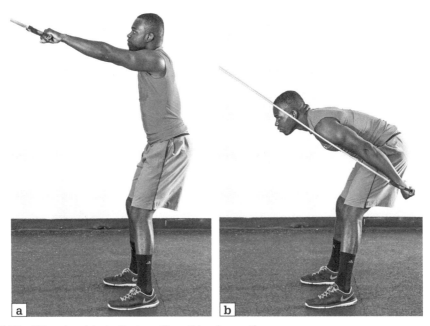

FIGURE 4.33 BP swim: *(a)* starting position; *(b)* swim motion.

BP High-to-Low Chop

Details and Benefits

- Natural progression to all planks, push-ups, and rotation with and without pivot
- Excellent fundamental exercise for the diagonal anterior and posterior core
- Useful in all sports that involve swinging an implement, such as baseball and golf, as well as throws and downward striking in combat sports

Starting Position

- Set the loading point as high as possible, well above the head.
- Hold one handle in both hands (i.e., hold the handle in the right hand and wrap the left hand over the right hand).
- Turn to the left so the loading point is to your right and above your head.
- Keep your knees slightly bent with your arms straight and in front of you.

Movement

- Keeping the core stiff, plant the right leg and rotate the right hip.
- Allow the body to rotate and the hands to come toward the loading point (figure 4.34a).
- As an option, allow a slight left-foot pivot to help with right-hip internal rotation. Do not allow the right ankle and knee to rotate to the loading side (no lateral rotation).
- Once your hands are at the top of the movement, perform a diagonal downward chopping motion.
- When the handles are halfway down (about chest level), shift your weight to the left foot with the toes pointing straight ahead and continue to chop down and across until the hands are outside and below the left hip (figure 4.34b).
- If needed, allow a slight right-foot pivot to finish the chop.
- Repeat the sequence.
- Perform on both sides of the body.

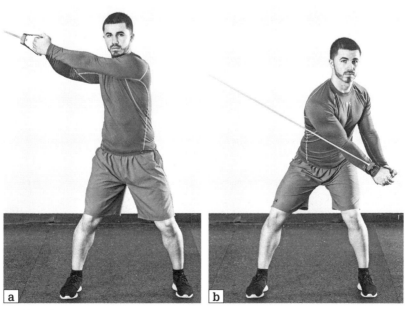

FIGURE 4.34 BP high-to-low chop: *(a)* high; *(b)* low.

BP Low-to-High Chop

Details and Benefits

- Natural progression to rotation with and without pivot as well as all lunging and chopping progressions
- Excellent fundamental exercise for the anterior and diagonal posterior musculature, especially the glutes
- Useful for all sports that involve changing directions and swinging an implement, such as tennis and baseball, as well as clinching and throws in combat sports

Starting Position

- Set the loading point as low as possible.
- Hold one handle in both hands (i.e., hold the handle with the right hand and wrap the left hand over the right hand).
- Turn to the left so the loading point is to your right and below your knees.
- Keep your knees slightly bent with your arms straight and in front of you.

Movement

- Keeping the core stiff, plant the right leg and rotate the right hip. Slightly hinging the hip to lean down, allow the body to rotate and the hands to come down toward the loading point (figure 4.35a). Allow a slight left-foot pivot to help with right-hip internal rotation. Do not allow the right ankle and knee to rotate to the loading side (no lateral rotation).
- Once your hands are at the bottom of the movement, perform a diagonal and upward reverse chopping motion until the hands are high and to the left of the left shoulder (figure 4.35b). Complete the movement perfectly centered between both feet and hands in front of the body with arms extended.
- Repeat the sequence.
- Perform on both sides of the body.

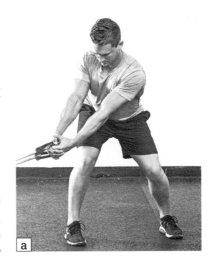

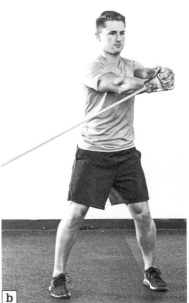

FIGURE 4.35 BP low-to-high chop: (a) low; (b) high.

BP Short Rotation (10 to 2 O'Clock)

Details and Benefits

- Natural progression from rotation with and without pivot and all planks and push-ups
- Fundamental exercise for rotational core stiffness
- Popular with combat and throwing athletes as well as those who swing implements

Starting Position

- Set the loading point at about chest-height.
- Hold one handle in both hands (i.e., hold the handle with the right hand and wrap the left hand over the right hand).
- Turn to the left so the loading point is to your right.
- Keep your knees slightly bent with the arms straight and in front of you (12 o'clock).

Movement

- Keeping the core stiff, perform short rotations to the left (10 o'clock; figure 4.36a) and right (2 o'clock; figure 4.36b) without allowing the hips to move.
- Repeat on both sides of the body.

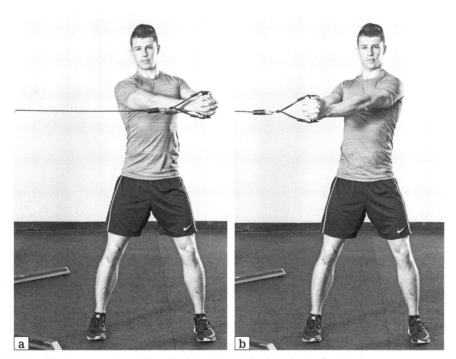

FIGURE 4.36 BP short rotation (10 to 2 o'clock): *(a)* 10 o'clock; *(b)* 2 o'clock.

BP Pulsating Backswing

Details and Benefits

- Natural progression to all high-to-low chops, push-ups, and rotation with and without pivot
- Unique exercise that develops the hips and core strength and flexibility needed for rotational mechanics
- Useful in all sports involving swinging an implement, such as baseball and golf, especially in the backswing

Starting Position

- Set the loading point as high as possible, well above the head.
- Hold one handle in both hands (i.e., hold the handle in the left hand and wrap the right hand over the left hand).
- Turn to the left so the loading point is to your right and above your head, the band or cable is over your head, and the handle is high and to the left (figure 4.37a).
- You should be in the backswing position that your sport requires.

Movement

- Keeping the core stiff, plant the left leg and internally rotate the left hip, allowing the load you take you deeper into the backswing.
- Allow the body to rotate and the hands to come toward the loading point (figure 4.37b), keeping perfect backswing mechanics for your sport.
- Pulsate through a short range of motion (about 10 in. [25 cm]) back and forth.
- Feel your core stiffen, your left hip internally rotate, and your backswing range of motion improve.
- Perform on both sides of the body.

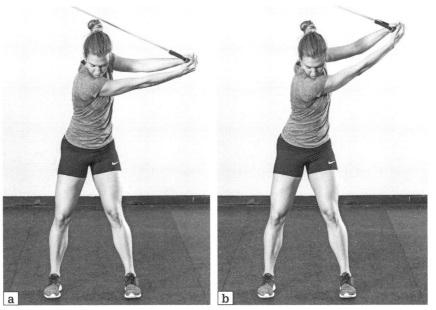

FIGURE 4.37 BP pulsating backswing: *(a)* starting position; *(b)* hands move toward loading point.

BP Push–Pull

Details and Benefits

- Natural progression from rotation with and without pivot and all standing horizontal pressing and rowing progressions
- Fundamental dual-cable exercise for rotational core stiffness and shoulder stability
- Popular with runners, combative athletes and those who swing implements

Starting Position

- Choose a dual-cable system that has two opposing loading points about 8 to 10 feet (2.5-3 m) apart. If a dual-cable system isn't available, this exercise may be done with two separate bands and partner assistance.
- Set the loading points at about chest-height.
- Hold one handle from each cable column in each hand.
- Facing the cable machine, turn to your left and assume a split-stance position while facing the right cable so the right arm is extended and the left hand is next to the chest, ready to press (figure 4.38a).

Movement

- Keeping the core stiff, simultaneously row with the right hand and press with the left hand (figure 4.38b).
- Repeat, simultaneously pushing and pulling.
- Repeat on both sides of the body, switching foot positions.

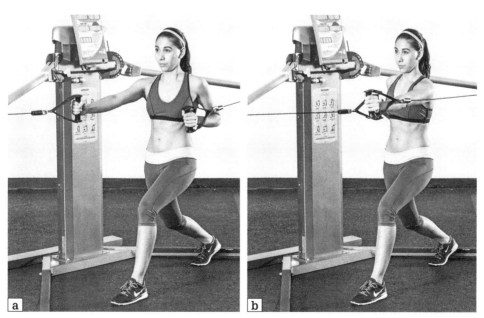

FIGURE 4.38 BP push–pull: (a) starting position; (b) row with right hand and press with left hand.

Dumbbells and Kettlebells

Once body weight and bands or cables are mastered, dumbbells (DB) and kettlebells (KB) are the equipment of choice to externally load any functional training exercise. Because they allow you to load each hand and perform exercises on the right side and left side, they can address muscular imbalances easily and naturally. The ability to use heavy or light loads allows you to focus on any quality you desire, from heavy strength work to light endurance work and everything in between. Even asymmetrical or unilateral loading can be easily addressed by carrying the load only in one hand. Chapter 1 provided information on where to obtain the best dumbbell and kettlebell products for functional training.

DB or KB Squat

Details and Benefits

- This is a foundational exercise that develops the core and lower body.
- It's an excellent way to add intensity to the bodyweight double-leg squat without directly placing a load on the spine (as in the barbell squat).
- Many versions and carrying positions are available; the basic shoulder-carry variation is described here.

Starting Position

- Stand tall with feet facing forward and shoulder-width apart.
- Hold a dumbbell or kettlebell in each hand at shoulder-height (figure 4.39a).
- Use the neutral position (i.e., palms facing in) to hold the dumbbells or kettlebells.

Movement

- Keeping your core stiff and holding the dumbbells or kettlebells in place, squat down to the parallel position (figure 4.39b).
- Stand up to return to the starting position.
- Repeat the squatting motion.

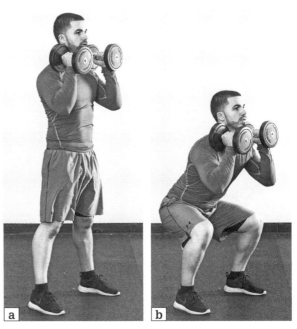

FIGURE 4.39 DB or KB squat: *(a)* starting position; *(b)* squat.

KB Single-Arm Swing

Details and Benefits

- Natural progression from and complement to all deadlift and squat progressions
- Excellent exercise to develop the dynamic extension of the ankles, knees, and hips used in jumping
- Popular with all jumping athletes

Starting Position

- Hold the kettlebell in the right hand, with the arm straight in front of the body and palm facing the body.
- Hinge at the hips with a straight back and with knees slightly flexed and feet facing forward, shoulder-width apart (figure 4.40a).

Movement

- Quickly extend the entire body to propel the kettlebell up in a circular path until the kettlebell is about shoulder-height with the right arm extended in front of you (figure 4.40b).
- Allow the kettlebell to travel down the same path it took up. Decelerate at the bottom of the swing and repeat the extension movement.
- Repeat on both sides.

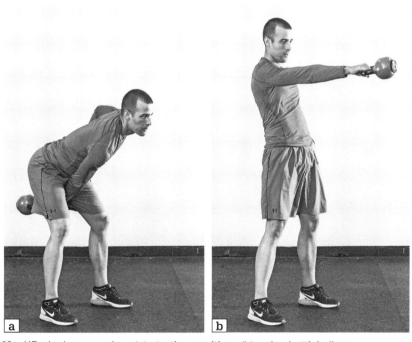

FIGURE 4.40   KB single-arm swing: *(a)* starting position; *(b)* swing kettlebell up.

DB or KB Single-Leg RDL (Romanian Deadlift)

Details and Benefits

- Natural progression from and complement to the single-leg CLA anterior reach and all BP staggered-stance rowing and deadlift progressions
- Excellent for developing strong hamstrings and glutes and decelerating mechanics
- Popular with athletes who require strong low positions and low deceleration and change-of-direction capabilities

Starting Position

- Hold the weight in the right hand, with the arm extended and hanging in front of the body, palm facing in.
- Balance on the left leg, with the left knee slightly flexed and the right leg back and off the ground (figure 4.41a).

Movement

- Stabilizing the single-leg position, hinge at the left hip until the core is almost parallel to the ground or until you feel a comfortable stretch in the left hamstring.
- Keeping the back straight throughout the entire movement, allow the arm to remain vertical at all times (figure 4.41b).
- Extend the hip to return to the starting position.
- Repeat the hip-flexing motion and perform on both sides of the body.

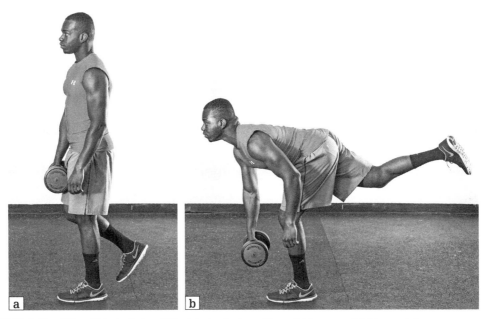

FIGURE 4.41 DB or KB single-leg RDL: *(a)* starting position; *(b)* lower weight toward floor.

DB or KB Lunge

Details and Benefits

- Intermediate to advanced progression once the bodyweight alternating lunge is mastered
- Excellent lower-body and core exercise that targets the hips and core
- Popular with combat athletes and field and court athletes, such as soccer and tennis players

Starting Position

- Stand up straight, feet pointing forward about shoulder-width apart.
- Hold a dumbbell or kettlebell in each hand. Hands are in front of you in the shoulder carry position—the position used right before performing a neutral-grip overhead press (figure 4.42a).

Movement

- Keeping your back straight, take a big step forward with the right leg.
- As the right foot lands, sink into a deep lunge or split-squat position (figure 4.42b).
- Push off the right foot to return to the starting position.
- Repeat on the left side and continue the alternating pattern.

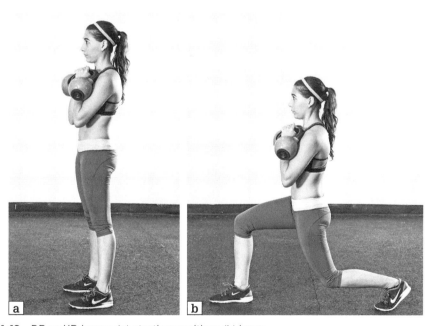

FIGURE 4.42 DB or KB lunge: *(a)* starting position; *(b)* lunge.

DB or KB Front Reaching Lunge

Details and Benefits

- Natural progression from and complement to the bodyweight alternating lunge and the BP staggered-stance deadlift and compound row progressions
- Excellent for strengthening the back, hips, and hamstrings with minimal knee involvement
- Popular with athletes who use low positions, such as wrestlers, and athletes who decelerate to change directions, such as tennis players and receivers

Starting Position

- Stand up tall with dumbbells or kettlebells in both hands (figure 4.43a).
- Arms are at the sides, palms facing in.
- Feet are hip-width apart.

Movement

- Take a big step with the left foot and land in a split stance. Your step should be long enough to keep the left knee above the ankle and the right knee behind the vertical shoulder–hip line. The right heel should be off the ground.
- As your left foot lands, keep your core tight. Flex your hips and allow the dumbbells or kettlebells to reach to the sides of the left foot (figure 4.43b). Go as low as your left hamstring flexibility will allow.
- Once you reach the bottom of the movement, push off the left foot and use your left hamstrings and glutes to extend the body and step back to the starting position.
- Repeat on the other side.

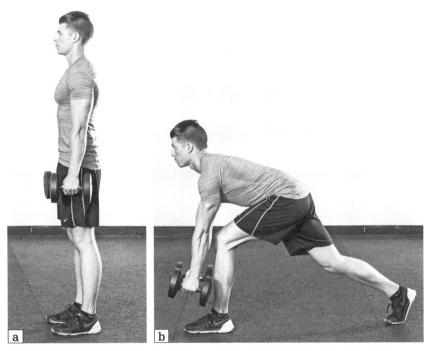

FIGURE 4.43 DB or KB front reaching lunge: *(a)* starting position; *(b)* lunge and reach.

DB or KB Lateral Reaching Lunge

Details and Benefits

- Natural progression from and complement to all single-leg progressions and the BP low-to-high chop
- Excellent exercise to develop rotational stability and flexibility of the external rotators of the hips as well as to strengthen the diagonal posterior musculature
- Especially good for unilateral glute activity and external hip rotators
- Uses minimal knee flexion, reducing wear and tear on the knees, while strengthening the hips and enhancing changes of direction; great progression for athletes who have knee issues
- Popular with athletes who need fast changes of direction (e.g., tennis and soccer players) as well as athletes who swing implements (e.g., batting, golfing)

Starting Position

- Stand tall with dumbbells or kettlebells in both hands (figure 4.44a).
- Arms are at the sides, palms facing in.
- Feet are hip-width apart.

Movement

- Take a big step to the left and land in a wide stance that is approximately double your shoulder-width.
- As your left foot lands, hinge your hips, allowing them to move back and flex.
- Flex your left knee, but minimize the flexion so your left shin is vertical and in line with the left ankle (figure 4.44b).

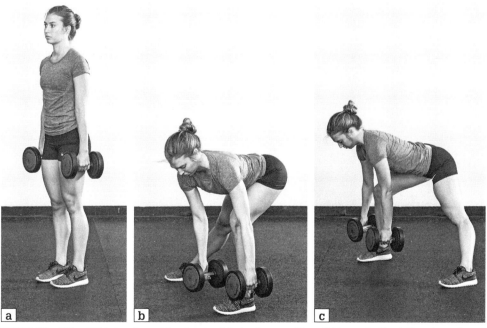

FIGURE 4.44   DB or KB lateral reaching lunge: (a) starting position; (b) lunge to the left and reach weights to foot; (c) lunge to the right and reach weights to foot.

- Keeping your back straight, continue to hinge the hips and reach the dumbbells or kettlebells to each side of the left foot.
- Once you reach the bottom of the movement, push off the left foot, using your left hamstring and glute to extend the body and step back to the starting position.
- Repeat on the other side (figure 4.44c).

DB or KB Rotating Reaching Lunge

Details and Benefits

- Natural progression from and complement to the rotational single-leg squat, all single-leg progressions, the BP low-to-high chop, and all reaching lunge progressions
- Excellent exercise to develop rotational stability and flexibility of the hips as well as to strengthen the diagonal posterior musculature, especially the glutes
- Uses minimal knee flexion, reducing wear and tear on the knees; great progression for athletes who have knee issues
- Popular with athletes who need fast opening steps and changes of direction

Starting Position

- Stand tall with dumbbells or kettlebells in both hands (figure 4.45a).
- Arms are at the sides, palms facing in.
- Feet are hip-width apart.

Movement

- Imagine you're standing in the middle of a square and take a big step (approximately double shoulder-width) to the right-rear corner.

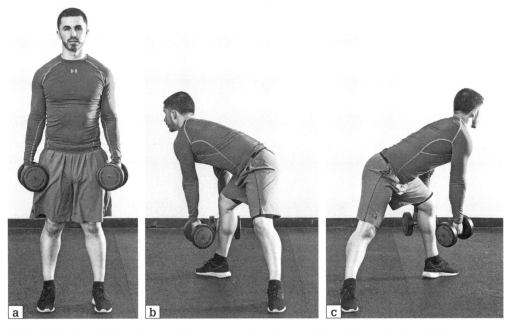

FIGURE 4.45 DB or KB rotating reaching lunge: *(a)* starting position; *(b)* lunge to the right rear and reach weights to foot; *(c)* lunge to the left and reach weights to foot.

- Land in a wide stance with the left foot facing forward and the right foot facing the right-rear corner of the imaginary square.

- As your right foot lands, move your hips toward the right foot, hinge the hips, and flex your right knee so that the right shin is vertical and over the right ankle (figure 4.45b).

- Keeping your back straight and minimizing right-knee flexion, continue to flex the right hip and reach each dumbbell to each side of the right foot. Reach as far as the right hamstring will allow.

- Once you reach the bottom of the movement, push off the right foot using your right hamstring, glute, and paraspinal muscles to extend the body and step back to the starting position.

- Repeat on the other side (figure 4.45c).

DB or KB Staggered-Stance Bent-Over Single-Arm Row

Details and Benefits

- Natural progression from and complement to the single-leg CLA anterior reach and all BP staggered-stance rowing and deadlift progressions

- Excellent for developing strong hamstrings, glutes, and back muscles

- Popular with athletes who require strong hamstrings for running and lifting, such as combat, field, and court athletes

Starting Position

- Hold the weight in the right hand using a neutral grip with the arms extended by your side.

- Stand in a split stance with the left leg forward and the knee over the ankle. The right leg is back, knee bent and behind the vertical shoulder–hip line, feet facing forward, and the leg stable on the ball of the foot.

- Hinge at the hips until the core is almost parallel to the ground or until you feel a comfortable stretch in the left hamstring.

- Keep the back straight throughout the entire movement and keep the right arm vertical at all times (figure 4.46a).

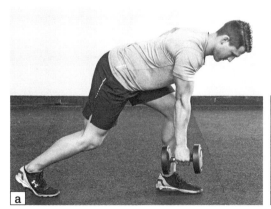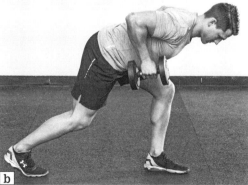

FIGURE 4.46   DB or KB staggered-stance bent-over single-arm row: *(a)* starting position; *(b)* row.

Movement

- Keeping the split-stance, bent-over position stable, pull the right hand in a rowing motion to the right side of the rib cage (figure 4.46b).
- Return the arm to the starting position and repeat the rowing motion.
- Perform on both sides of the body.
- For more advanced hip training, this exercise can be performed on one leg.

DB or KB Overhead Press

Details and Benefits

- Natural progression from and complement to all BP pressing progressions and push-up progressions
- Excellent exercise to develop shoulder strength and stability and core strength
- Popular with athletes who need total-body strength and shoulder flexibility

Starting Position

- Stand up tall, feet facing forward and shoulder-width apart. Keep the core tight throughout the movement.
- Hold a dumbbell or kettlebell in each hand and at shoulder-height, palms facing each other (figure 4.47a).

Movement

- Although the alternating pattern is explained here, this exercise can be performed simultaneously with both arms.
- Perform an overhead press with the right hand while keeping the left hand at the shoulder line (figure 4.47b).
- Bring the right hand down to the right shoulder while pressing the left hand overhead.
- You may use slight lateral flexion of the body to accommodate reduced range of motion at the shoulders, but keep the core tight and engaged at all times.
- Repeat the alternating pressing action.

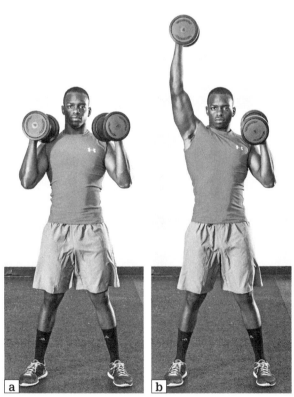

FIGURE 4.47 DB or KB overhead press: *(a)* starting position; *(b)* overhead press.

DB or KB Lateral Overhead Press

This exercise can be performed with the arms out to the sides and palms facing forward, moving the arms simultaneously (figure 4.48). This version provides greater shoulder involvement and is popular with bodybuilders. Single-arm variations and additional lateral movement of the body also allow easier vertical pressing if shoulder flexibility is a concern.

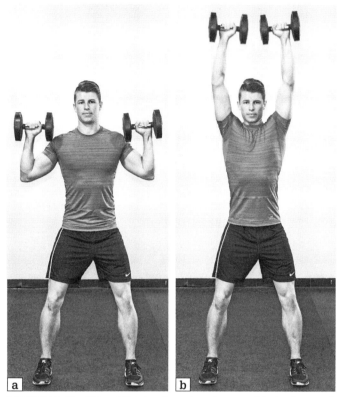

FIGURE 4.48   DB or KB lateral overhead press: *(a)* starting position; *(b)* overhead press.

DB or KB Overhead Y Press

Details and Benefits
- Natural progression from and complement to all BP pressing progressions and push-up progressions
- Excellent exercise to develop shoulder strength and stability and core strength
- Popular with athletes who need total-body strength and shoulder flexibility

Starting Position
- Stand up tall, feet facing forward and shoulder-width apart. Keep the core tight throughout the movement.
- Hold a dumbbell or kettlebell in each hand outside the shoulders, palms facing forward (figure 4.49*a*).

Movement
- Perform a diagonal (up and out) overhead press with the right hand while keeping the left hand outside the left shoulder line (figure 4.49*b*).
- Bring the right hand down to the outside of the right shoulder while diagonally pressing the left hand.
- Keep the core tight and engaged at all times.
- Repeat the alternating Y-pressing action.

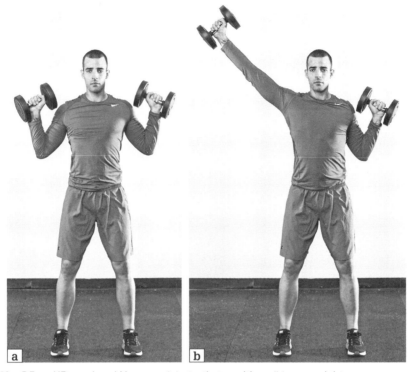

FIGURE 4.49 DB or KB overhead Y press: *(a)* starting position; *(b)* press right.

DB or KB Cross Overhead Press

Details and Benefits

- Natural progression from and complement to all BP pressing progressions, push-up progressions, and rotational progressions

- Excellent exercise to develop shoulder strength and stability, hip internal rotation, and core strength seen in the backswing and follow-through of swings

- Popular with athletes who swing implements, such as in batting and golfing

Starting Position

- Stand up tall, feet facing forward and shoulder-width apart.

- Hold a dumbbell or kettlebell in each hand at shoulder-height, palms facing each other (figure 4.50a).

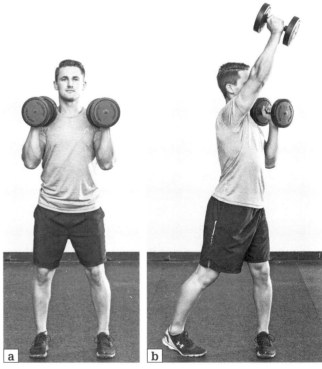

FIGURE 4.50 DB or KB cross overhead press: *(a)* starting position; *(b)* overhead press.

Movement

- Perform an overhead press with the right hand as you plant the left foot and pivot the right foot, internally rotating the left hip (figure 4.50b). Avoid external rotation of the left knee and ankle.
- Bring the right hand down to the right shoulder while turning left to the starting position.
- Smoothly transition through the starting point and perform the left-hand cross overhead press to the right side, while pivoting on the left foot.
- Repeat the rotational pressing action.

DB High Cross Punch

The cross overhead press without a pivot is also called the *high cross punch*. It is popular with combat athletes to develop shoulder strength and core stiffness. Usually it is performed with dumbbells. Stand up tall, feet facing forward and shoulder-width apart. Hold a dumbbell in each hand at shoulder-height, palms facing each other. Keeping your core and lower body stiff, punch with the right hand across the body and up so the dumbbell is high and outside the left shoulder (figure 4.51). Bring the right hand back and perform a high cross punch with the left hand. Repeat the pattern.

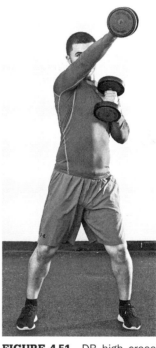

FIGURE 4.51 DB high cross punch.

DB or KB Biceps Curl

Details and Benefits

- Natural progression from and complement to all DB or KB carry and upright rowing progressions
- Excellent exercise to develop arm, shoulder, and core strength
- Popular with combat athletes and athletes in contact sports

Starting Position

- Stand up tall, feet facing forward and shoulder-width apart. Keep the core tight throughout the movement.
- Hold a dumbbell or kettlebell in each hand down by your sides, palms facing forward.

Movement

- Although the alternating pattern is explained here, this exercise can be performed simultaneously with both arms.

- Perform a curl with the right hand while keeping the left hand by your side (figure 4.52*a*).

- Bring the right hand down to the right side while performing a curl with the left hand (figure 4.52*b*).

- You may use slight core movement if needed for balance, but keep the core tight and engaged at all times.

- Repeat the alternating curling action.

- This exercise can be performed on one leg to add single-leg, 7-frame stability while still developing arm strength.

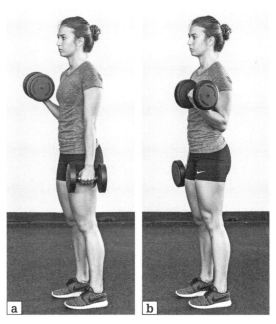

FIGURE 4.52 DB or KB biceps curl: *(a)* curl right; *(b)* curl left.

Running Curl

The running curl can be performed with more of a running action, and it's an awesome addition to a running program. To perform the running curl, stand with your knees slightly flexed, core tight, and arms at your sides with palms facing your body. Flex your right arm until it's at 90 degrees and the dumbbell is in front of you. At the same time, allow your left arm to go back for counterbalance (figure 4.53). Perform a running motion with your arms without allowing the core or lower body to move.

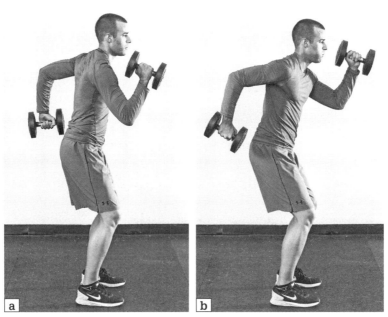

FIGURE 4.53 Running curl: *(a)* right-arm flex; *(b)* left-arm flex.

DB or KB Upright Row

Details and Benefits

- Natural progression from and complement to all low-to-high rowing and biceps curl progressions
- Excellent exercise to develop arm, shoulder, and core strength
- Popular with runners, combat athletes, and athletes in contact sports

Starting Position

- Stand up tall, feet facing forward and shoulder-width apart. Keep the core tight throughout the movement.
- Slightly flex forward so the dumbbells or kettlebells can move up without contacting the body.
- Hold a dumbbell or kettlebell in each hand down in front of you, palms facing your body.

Movement

- Although the alternating pattern is explained here, this exercise can be performed simultaneously with both arms.
- Perform an upright row with the right hand until the dumbbell or kettlebell is at about chest-height. At the same time, keep the left hand down in front of you (figure 4.54a).
- Bring the right hand down in front of you while performing an upright row with the left hand until the dumbbell or kettlebell is at about chest-height (figure 4.54b).
- You may use slight rotational shoulder and core movement as needed for balance, but keep the core tight and engaged at all times.
- Repeat the alternating rowing action.
- This exercise can be performed on one leg to add single-leg, 7-frame stability while still developing arm strength.

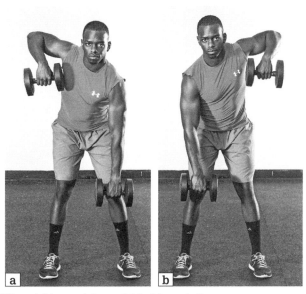

FIGURE 4.54 DB or KB upright row: *(a)* row right; *(b)* row left.

DB or KB Cross Uppercut

Details and Benefits

- Natural progression from and complement to all DB or KB curl, carry, and upright rowing progressions
- Excellent exercise to develop arm, shoulder, and core strength
- Popular with runners, combat athletes, and athletes in contact sports

Starting Position

- Stand up tall, feet facing forward and shoulder-width apart. Keep the core tight throughout the movement.
- Hold a dumbbell or kettlebell in each hand down by your sides, palms facing the body.

Movement

- Flex the right arm and perform a cross uppercut with the right arm across the body and to the left while pivoting on the right foot until the dumbbell or kettlebell is in line and to the outside of the left shoulder (figure 4.55a).
- Bring the right hand down to the right side while keeping the right elbow flexed. At the same time, perform a cross uppercut with the left arm across the body and to the right while pivoting on the left foot until the dumbbell or kettlebell is in line and to the outside of the right shoulder (figure 4.55b).
- Keep the core tight and engaged at all times.
- Repeat the alternating cross uppercut.

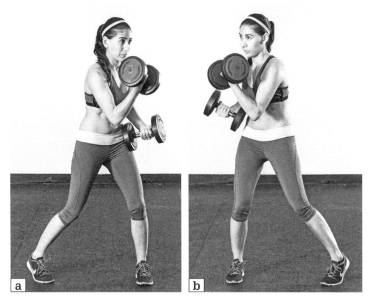

FIGURE 4.55 DB or KB cross uppercut: *(a)* uppercut right; *(b)* uppercut left.

Modified Clinch Curl

The simultaneous DB or KB upper-cut is also called a *modified clinch curl*. Combat athletes use it to create a strong clinch (arm grappling from the standing position) and strong lifting mechanics. It looks like a form of a cheated curl. Stand with the dumbbells or kettlebells in your hands, with arms flexed about 90 degrees, hips hinging, back straight, and shoulders leaning forward as if you were going to pick up a box in front of you at hip-height (figure 4.56a). The bottom position can also be low as it will allow your forearms to rest on top of your thighs. Use the depth needed in the sports you are preparing for. Using your whole body, extend your body and curl both weights up until they are at shoulder-height (figure 4.56b). Return to the starting position and repeat.

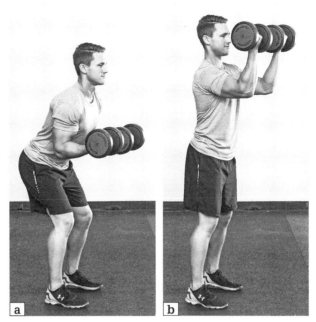

FIGURE 4.56   Modified clinch curl: *(a)* starting position; *(b)* curl both weights.

DB Horizontal Fly Rotation

Details and Benefits

- Natural progression from and complement to X-ups, BP rotations, BP flys, and BP presses
- Unique exercise that develops core stability during rotational movements
- Popular with golfers, baseball players, and board athletes who use the upper body as a long lever to facilitate lower-body movement and total-body rotational power

Starting Position

- Stand up tall, feet facing forward and shoulder-width apart, knees slightly flexed.
- Hold a dumbbell up and out in each hand at shoulder-height in a T-position; elbows are slightly flexed and palms are facing forward (figure 4.57a).

Movement

- Keeping your core stiff and feet firmly planted, rotate your body to the right, bringing the left arm forward and right arm back (figure 4.57b). The hips and shoulders should always rotate together with a super stiff core and slight flexion at the knees.
- When the right rotation is complete, rotate to the left, bringing the right arm forward and left arm back, smoothly transitioning through the starting point all the way through the end of the right rotation.
- Repeat the rotation to both sides.

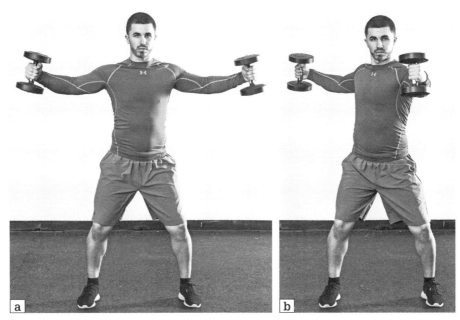

FIGURE 4.57 DB horizontal fly rotation: *(a)* starting position; *(b)* rotate to the right.

DB Single-Arm Diagonal Fly Rotation

Details and Benefits

- Natural progression from and complement to the BP high-to-low and low-to-high chops, MB short diagonal chop (chapter 5), DB horizontal fly rotation, and DB or KB lateral reaching lunge
- Unique exercise that develops core stability for rotational movements and decelerating throwing motion
- Popular with golfers, baseball players, and board athletes who use the upper body as a long lever to facilitate lower-body movement and total-body rotational power

Starting Position

- Stand up tall, feet facing forward and shoulder-width apart, knees slightly flexed and feet firmly planted.
- Hold a dumbbell in the right hand to the right side of the body and above the head, allowing the shoulders to rotate to the right, as if getting ready to throw a ball (figure 4.58a).

Movement

- Keeping your core stiff, make a diagonal throwing motion with the right hand, bringing the right hand to the left side of the body between the left hip and left knee (figure 4.58b).
- The hips and shoulders should always rotate together with good internal rotation of the left hip and a slight pivot on the right foot can be used to facilitate left hip internal rotation. There should be no rotation at the left knee or ankle during the entire movement.
- At the end of the rotation, bring the right hand back to the starting position.
- Repeat the throwing motion and perform on both sides of the body.

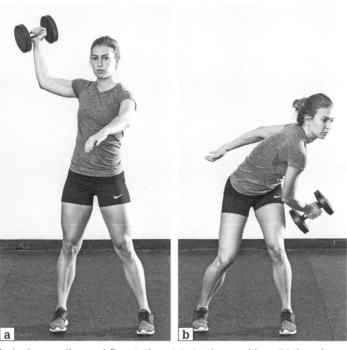

FIGURE 4.58 DB single-arm diagonal fly rotation: *(a)* starting position; *(b)* throwing motion.

DB or KB Carry

Details and Benefits

- Foundational exercise that develops the core stiffness needed to perform any standing exercise or activity, especially if it involves carrying an object
- Develops the diaphragmatic breathing and dynamic core stiffness needed in contact sports, especially grappling combat sports

Starting Position

- Stand up tall with a weight in each hands (figure 4.59).
- Bend the elbows until they are flexed to about 90 degrees.

Movement

- Keeping your core stiff, hold the dumbbells or kettlebells in place.
- Although this exercise can be performed stationary for time, the better option is to perform the carry while walking for time.

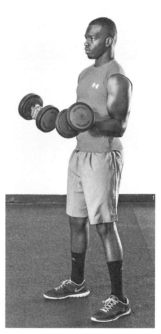

FIGURE 4.59 DB or KB carry.

Conclusion

The modalities and exercises in this chapter are the most versatile and essential to functional training. Any athlete who trains and masters the evaluation exercises in chapter 3 plus the exercises here will be well on her way to being ready to perform at her best, regardless of level. The modalities and exercises in chapter 5 will add even more diversity to your functional training program.

CHAPTER 5

The Supporting Cast

Chapter 4 provided the main exercises needed for a functional training program, and now this chapter provides the rest of the exercises to add diversity, effectiveness, and fun to your training. This chapter includes medicine ball core and power applications, stability ball core and rotational exercises, exercises using industry toys for agility and power training, and even some traditional exercises for hypertrophy that illustrate the effectiveness of IHP's hybrid training. The exercises follow the same format as in chapter 4: photos to illustrate the movement, some details on the exercise, and instructions to support the proper execution of the exercise.

Remember, pain and control are the two best indicators of how appropriate the progression is: No pain and good form almost always mean the progression is appropriate. If in doubt, start conservatively and add repetitions to increase volume. Volume is the best variable to increase, especially at the beginning of training. Volume allows learning, reinforces good patterns, helps to eliminate imbalances, provides strength, and burns calories, which is important to athletes trying to lose excess fat. Increasing load and speed come once the movement is automatic and can be performed correctly without any thought to form.

Medicine Balls

Medicine balls (MB) have been used by combat and track athletes for many years. Their original use focused on core exercise and throws. With the increased popularity of core exercises and functional training, medicine balls underwent an evolution. They now come in many shapes and sizes, some with handles, ropes, and bar attachments. Where the original medicine balls weighed a few pounds, now they can weigh over 40 pounds (18 kg), capable of providing high-level strength training for some people.

MB Wood Chop

Details and Benefits

- Basic total-body progression to add to the bodyweight double-leg squat (chapter 3)
- Arguably the best total-body medicine ball exercise
- Can be used for warming up the whole body, evaluating movement, and improving vertical jumps

Starting Position

- Stand upright, feet pointing forward and about shoulder-width apart.
- Hold the medicine ball in both hands overhead, with the elbows extended as far as comfortably possible (figure 5.1a).

Movement

- Keeping your back straight, squat down, hinging at the hips and flexing your knees and ankles while performing a downward semicircular chop with the ball (figure 5.1b).
- Stop when your upper leg is parallel to the ground, the ball is close to the ground, and your elbows are inside your thighs.
- Return to the starting position and repeat the chopping motion in the same direction.

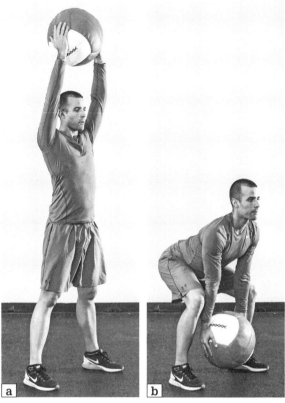

FIGURE 5.1 MB wood chop: (a) starting position; (b) squat and chop.

MB Short Wood Chop

The wood chop can be performed as a short wood chop without the squatting motion. Plant your feet with knees slightly bent and the core upright and stiff. Hold the medicine ball in front of you with arms extended. Imagine there is a rectangle in front of you from your head to your hips and from shoulder to shoulder. Without moving your core or lower body, make a vertical chopping motion from the top to the bottom of the rectangle (figure 5.2). Repeat the chopping motion as fast as possible without moving the core.

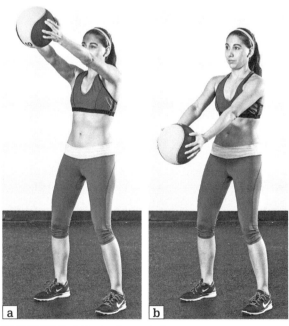

FIGURE 5.2 MB short wood chop.

MB Diagonal Chop

Details and Benefits

- Basic total-body progression from the MB wood chop and all squatting progressions as well as a perfect complement to the BP low-to-high chop
- Can be used for warming up the whole body, evaluating movement, and improving lateral changes in direction and swinging mechanics

Starting Position

- Stand upright, feet pointing forward and about shoulder-width apart.
- Hold the medicine ball in both hands overhead to the right side of the body, with the arms extended and the left foot pivoted inward (internally rotating right hip) (figure 5.3a).

Movement

- Keeping your back straight, squat down and rotate to the left, hinging at the hips and flexing your knees and ankles.
- As you reach the middle of the rotation (facing forward), internally rotate at the left hip, pivoting your right foot in, and perform a downward diagonal chop with the ball (figure 5.3b).
- Stop when the ball is outside your left knee.
- Return to the starting position and repeat the diagonal chopping motion.
- Perform to both sides of the body.

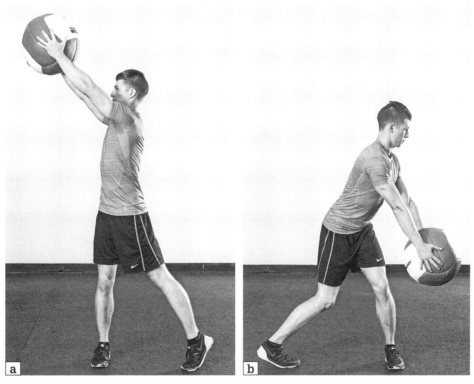

FIGURE 5.3 MB diagonal chop: *(a)* starting position; *(b)* low chop.

MB Short Diagonal Chop

The MB diagonal chop can be performed as a short diagonal chop without the squatting motion, just like the BP short rotation and the rotation without pivot. Plant your feet with the knees slightly bent and the core upright and stiff. Hold the medicine ball in front of you with arms extended. Imagine a rectangle in front of you from your head to your hips and from shoulder to shoulder. Without moving your core or lower body, make a chopping motion from the upper-right corner to the lower-left corner of the rectangle (figure 5.4). Repeat the chopping motion as fast as possible without moving the core. Perform the chopping motion to both sides of the body (i.e., upper left to lower right).

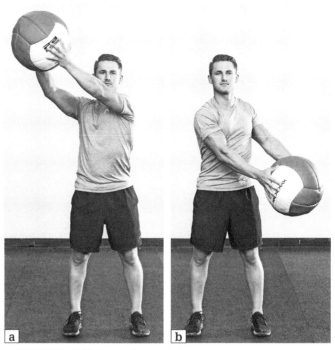

FIGURE 5.4 MB short diagonal chop.

MB ABC Squat

Details and Benefits

- Basic total-body progression that adds a multiplanar stimulus to all squatting progressions
- Perfect complement to a squat
- May be used to fix any hip deviations observed during squatting
- Popular with athletes who need multidirectional movement from a low squatting position, such as baseball catchers and volleyball players

Starting Position

- Stand with knees slightly flexed, feet pointing forward and about shoulder-width apart.
- Hold the medicine ball close to you at chest level with both hands.

Movement

- Keeping your back straight, squat down by hinging at the hips and flexing your knees and ankles while pushing the ball out in front of you (i.e., 12 o'clock; figure 5.5a).
- Stop when your upper legs are parallel to the ground.
- Return to the starting position.
- Squat down again, this time pushing the ball out to the right side of the body (i.e., 2 o'clock; figure 5.5b).
- Return to the starting position.

- Squat one last time, pushing the ball out to the left side of the body (i.e., 10 o'clock; figure 5.5c).
- Return to the starting position.
- Repeat the three-direction squat-and-push sequence (i.e., ABC pattern).

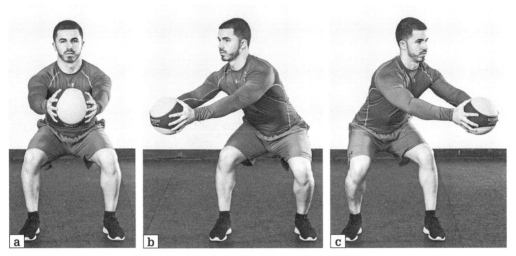

FIGURE 5.5   MB ABC squat: *(a)* 12 o'clock; *(b)* 2 o'clock; *(c)* 10 o'clock.

MB Lunge With Rotation

Details and Benefits

- Intermediate to advanced progression once the bodyweight alternating lunge and rotation with pivot (chapter 3) progressions are mastered.
- Excellent lower-body and rotational core exercise that targets the diagonal posterior and anterior musculature
- Popular with tennis players

Starting Position

- Stand up straight, feet pointing forward and about shoulder-width apart.
- Hold the medicine ball in both hands in front of you, with the elbows flexed (figure 5.6a).

Movement

- Keeping your back straight, take a big step forward with the right leg.
- As the right foot lands, sink into the lunge while rotating the ball and upper body to the right (figure 5.6b).

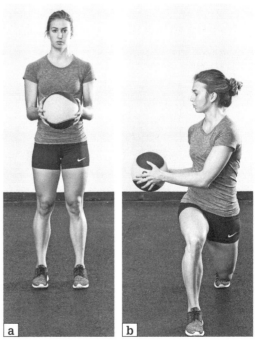

FIGURE 5.6   MB lunge with rotation: *(a)* starting position; *(b)* rotate to the right.

- Push off the right foot to return to the starting position.
- Repeat on the left side, rotating the ball and upper body to the left.
- Continue to alternate the lunge.

MB Single-Arm Push-Off

Details and Benefits

- Intermediate to advanced push-up progression of the bodyweight push-up, plank, and single-arm eccentrics; great lead-in to any single-arm plank or push-up variation
- Develops pushing power and the diagonal anterior core musculature used by combative athletes and football players

Starting Position

- Stabilize the body in a plank position with the right hand on the floor and the arm extended. The left hand is on top of a medicine ball with the arm flexed (figure 5.7a).
- Make sure your shoulders are parallel to the ground at all times.

Movement

- Flex the elbows to perform a push-up on the right side of the ball, keeping the core tight, the body straight, and the shoulders parallel to the ground at all times (figure 5.7b).
- Once the left elbow has flexed to 90 degrees, push up until the extended right arm lifts off the ground and the left arm performs a lock-out on the ball in the three-point position (figure 5.7c).
- Lower your body using only the left hand until the right arm touches the ground and proceed to lower into the two-arm push-up.
- Repeat the single-arm push-off on the left arm for desired repetitions.
- Perform on both arms.

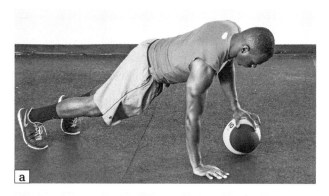

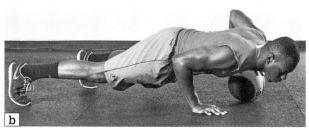

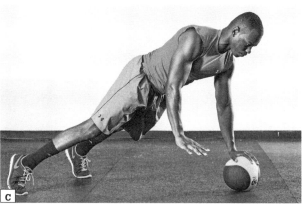

FIGURE 5.7 MB single-arm push-off: *(a)* starting position; *(b)* lower body to ground; *(c)* push up until right arm is off the ground and left arm is locked out.

MB Crossover Push-Up

Details and Benefits

- Intermediate to advanced push-up progression that follows the bodyweight push-up, plank, and MB single-arm push-off progression
- Develops pushing power and the diagonal anterior core musculature used by combative athletes and football players

Starting Position

- Stabilize the body in a plank position with the right hand on the floor and the arm extended. The left hand is on top of a medicine ball with the arm flexed.
- Make sure your shoulders are parallel to the ground at all times.

Movement

- Flex the elbows to perform a push-up on the right side of the ball, keeping the core tight, the body straight, and the shoulders parallel to the ground at all times (figure 5.8a).

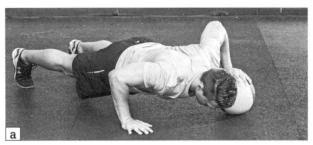

- Once the left elbow has flexed to 90 degrees, push up and place the right hand on the ball next to the left hand (figure 5.8b).
- Shift your weight to the left side of the ball and place your left hand on the floor to perform a push-up on the left side of the ball with the right hand on the ball (figure 5.8c).

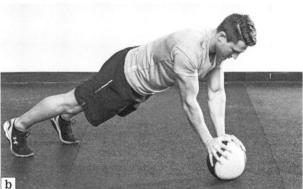

- Flex the elbows to perform a push-up until the right elbow has flexed to 90 degrees. Then push up and place the left hand next to the right hand on the ball.
- Shift your weight to the right side of the ball and place your right hand on the floor to perform a push-up on the right side of the ball with the left hand on the ball.
- Repeat the sequence.

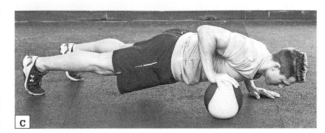

FIGURE 5.8 MB crossover push-up: (a) push-up on right side of ball; (b) both hands on ball; (c) push-up on left side of ball.

MB Rotation With Pivot

Details and Benefits

- Basic total-body progression from the body-weight rotation with pivot and the BP short rotation as well as a perfect complement to the BP low-to-high chop
- Can be used as for warming up the whole body, evaluating movement, and improving hip flexibility, lateral changes in direction, and swinging mechanics

Starting Position

- Stand upright, feet pointing forward and about shoulder-width apart.
- Hold the medicine ball in both hands in front of the body, with the elbows slightly flexed.

Movement

- Keeping your back straight, rotate to the left, internally rotating your left hip and pivoting your right foot without the left knee or ankle rotating outward (figure 5.9a).
- Stop when you can't internally rotate the left hip any farther.
- Rotate to the right, planting the right foot facing forward and pivoting on your left foot while internally rotating your right hip without the right knee or ankle rotating outward (figure 5.9b).
- Stop when you can't internally rotate the right hip any farther.
- Continue to perform side-to-side rotations with pivots.

MB Rotation Without Pivot

The MB rotation with pivot can be performed without pivots to create short rotations and greater core stiffness. Plant your feet with knees slightly bent and the core upright and stiff. Hold the ball in front of you with arms slightly flexed. Imagining you are a clock, hold the ball at 12 o'clock. Without moving your core or lower body, rotate your shoulders and move the ball to 10 o'clock. Rotating only the shoulders, move the ball to 2 o'clock. Continue the rotation from 10 to 2 o'clock without moving your core or lower body.

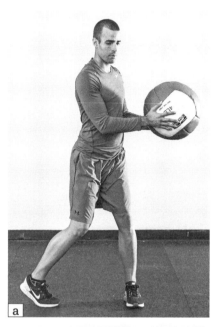

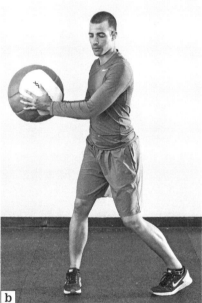

FIGURE 5.9 MB rotation with pivot: *(a)* rotate to the left; *(b)* rotate to the right.

MB Staggered-Stance CLA Incline Chest Throw

Details and Benefits

- This is a unique chest and rotational core progression that follows the DB or KB cross overhead press with pivot and BP presses (chapter 4).
- It develops the pushing and punching power used by combative athletes and track and field throwers, such as shot-putters. It also enhances the rotational power used by all throwing athletes.
- Use a ball with a live bounce if throwing from distance; use a ball with no bounce when throwing close to a wall, especially if in a busy gym.

Starting Position

- Stand sideways to a wall about 15 feet (5 m) away or closer if you are using a ball with no bounce.
- Stand with your feet shoulder-width apart and the left foot and shoulder closest to the wall, almost in a batting position.
- Hold the medicine ball with both hands to the right side of the chest, with the right elbow down and the palm on the ball (figure 5.10a).
- Use the left hand to hold the ball in place.

Movement

- Keeping the core tight, push off the right foot and take a step with the left foot, as if you were performing a batting motion.
- Simultaneously rotate left while using the right hand to push the medicine ball upward at a 45-degree angle (figure 5.10b).
- Finish the throw with a right-foot pivot, facing the wall in a long staggered stance.
- Catch the ball on the bounce and repeat.
- Perform to both sides of the body.

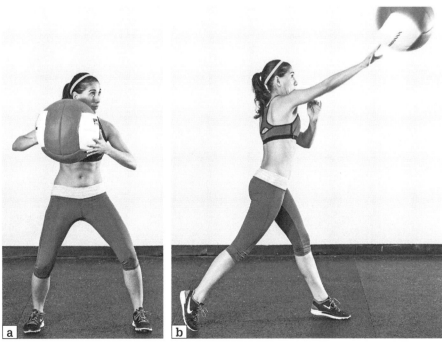

FIGURE 5.10 MB staggered-stance CLA incline chest throw: *(a)* starting position; *(b)* rotate left and push the medicine ball up at 45-degree angle.

MB Staggered-Stance CLA Straight Chest Throw

Details and Benefits

- This is a popular chest and rotational core progression that follows push-ups and cable presses.
- It develops the punching power used by combative athletes, as well as movements such as a stiff arm used in football. It also enhances the rotational power used by all throwing athletes.
- Use a ball with a live bounce if throwing from distance; use a ball with no bounce when throwing close to a wall, especially if in a busy gym.

Starting Position

- Stand sideways to a wall about 15 feet (5 m) away (or closer if you are using a ball with no bounce).
- Stand with your feet shoulder-width apart and the left foot and shoulder closest to the wall, almost in a batting position.
- Hold the medicine ball in both hands to the right side of the chest, with the right elbow up and forearm parallel to the ground (figure 5.11a).
- The right palm is on the ball and the left hand holds the ball in place.

Movement

- Keeping the core tight, push off the right foot and take a step with the left foot, as if you were performing a batting motion.
- Simultaneously rotate left while pushing the medicine ball with the right hand straight to the wall (figure 5.11b).
- Finish the throw with a right-foot pivot, facing the wall in a long staggered stance.
- Catch the ball on the bounce and repeat.
- Perform to both sides of the body.

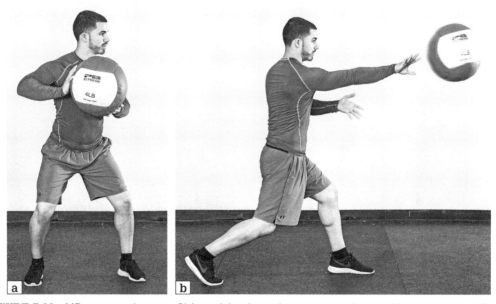

FIGURE 5.11 MB staggered-stance CLA straight chest throw: *(a)* starting position; *(b)* rotate left and push ball straight to the wall.

MB Staggered-Stance CLA Decline Chest Throw

Details and Benefits

- This is a basic chest and rotational core progression that follows push-ups and cable presses.
- It develops the downward pushing power used by combative athletes such as wrestlers.
- Use a ball with a live bounce if throwing from a distance; use a ball with no bounce when throwing close to a wall.

Starting Position

- Stand sideways to a wall about 5 feet (2 m) away (or closer if you are using a ball with no bounce), feet shoulder-width apart, with the right foot and shoulder closest to the wall.
- Hold the medicine ball with both hands to the left side of chest, with the left elbow up and forearm pointing down (figure 5.12a).
- The left palm is on the ball and the right hand holds the ball in place.

Movement

- Keeping the core tight, push off the left foot and take a step with the right foot.
- Simultaneously rotate right while using the left hand to push the medicine ball down at a 45-degree angle (figure 5.12b).
- Finish the throw with a left-foot pivot, facing the wall in a long staggered stance.
- Bounce the ball off the ground and wall and catch and repeat.
- Perform to both sides of the body.

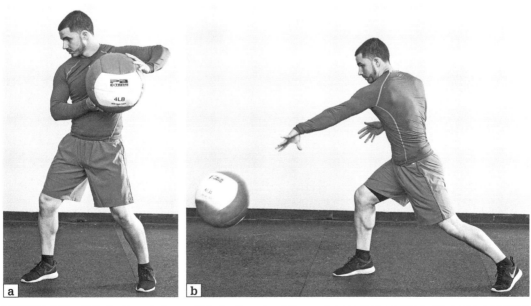

FIGURE 5.12 MB staggered-stance CLA decline chest throw: (a) starting position; (b) rotate and push ball down.

MB Overhead Slam

Details and Benefits

- This is an effective shoulder and core progression that follows any pulling or rowing, X-up, and knee-tuck progressions.
- It develops the throwing power used by many field athletes. It's also popular for the shoulder and core training of swimmers and combative athletes.
- Use a ball with a low bounce.

Starting Position

- Stand in a parallel stance with feet shoulder-width apart.
- Hold the medicine ball with both hands in front of you, arms extended.

Movement

- Keeping the core tight, bring the medicine ball overhead by fully extending the body (figure 5.13a).
- Slam the ball down about 2 to 3 feet (.5-1 m) in front of you (figure 5.13b).
- Be careful not to bounce the ball too close to you so as to avoid contact with the body. The ball should land far enough out that it does not hit your face when it rebounds.
- Catch the ball on the bounce and repeat. You can take a short step forward to catch the ball if necessary.
- Perform to both sides of the body.

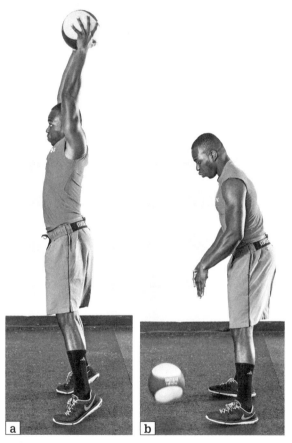

FIGURE 5.13 MB overhead slam: (a) bring ball overhead; (b) slam it to the ground.

MB Overhead Side-to-Side Slam

The MB overhead side-to-side slam variation is an intermediate shoulder, core, and rotational exercise. Like the MB overhead slam, this exercise develops the throwing power used by many field athletes and the rotational pivoting used in golf. Be sure to use a ball with a low bounce.

The starting position is the same as the MB overhead slam. Bring the medicine ball overhead by fully extending the body. Rotate to the right, pivoting on the left foot, and slam the ball down about a foot (30 cm) outside your right foot (figure 5.14a). Catch the ball on the rebound and then rotate to the left, pivoting with the right foot and slamming the ball down about a foot (30 cm) outside your left foot (figure 5.14b). Repeat on both sides. Be careful not to bounce the ball too close to you so as to avoid contact with the body, especially with the face.

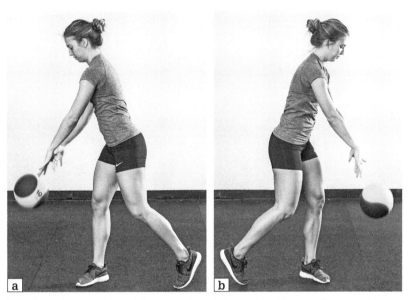

FIGURE 5.14 MB overhead side-to-side slam: *(a)* rotate to the right and throw ball down; *(b)* rotate to the left and throw ball down.

MB Rotational Throw: Perpendicular

Details and Benefits

- This is the fundamental medicine ball rotational power progression; it supplements all rotational training.
- It develops the rotational power used by many athletes in field and court sports, whether throwing or swinging an implement.
- Use a ball with a live bounce if throwing from distance; use a ball with no bounce when throwing close to a wall, especially if in a busy gym.

Starting Position

- Stand sideways to a wall about 15 feet (5 m) away (or closer if you are using a ball with no bounce), feet shoulder-width apart, with the left foot and shoulder closest to the wall, almost in a batting position.
- Hold the medicine ball with both hands in front of you, arms extended.

Movement

- Keeping the core tight and arms extended, rotate to the right to load the throw by planting the right foot and slightly pivoting the left foot (figure 5.15a). This action loads the right hip.
- Keeping the core tight, push off the right foot and take a step with the left foot, as if you were performing a batting motion (figure 5.15b).
- Finish the throw with a right-foot pivot, facing the wall in a long staggered stance.
- Retrieve the ball and repeat.
- Perform to both sides of the body.

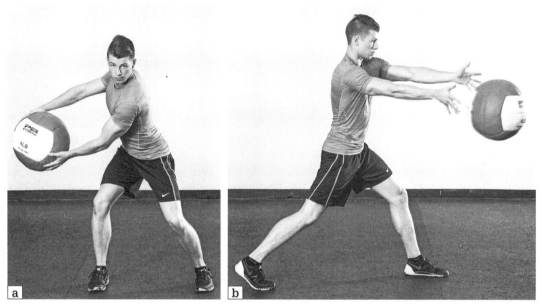

FIGURE 5.15 MB rotational throw: perpendicular: *(a)* rotate to the right; *(b)* rotate to the left and throw ball.

MB Reverse Scoop Throw

Details and Benefits

- This is an excellent progression to squatting and jumping exercises.
- It improves triple extension mechanics and vertical jumping.
- You can perform it in an open field with a partner (recommended) or against a wall close behind the body. I recommend an open field because bouncing a weighted medicine ball overhead and avoiding contact on the bounce takes some practice.
- A runaway heavy medicine ball can cause injury to anyone in the surrounding area. If you are going to use a wall rebound, use a ball with a soft bounce to limit its rolling and speed.

Starting Position

- Stand in a parallel stance with feet shoulder-width apart.
- Hold the medicine ball with both hands in front of you, arms extended.

Movement

- Keeping the arms extended and the core tight, perform a quarter squat and hinge at the hips to bring the ball between the legs and fore- arms between the thighs (figure 5.16a).

- Explode up and throw the ball backward at a 45-degree angle to get maximum height and dis- tance (figure 5.16b).

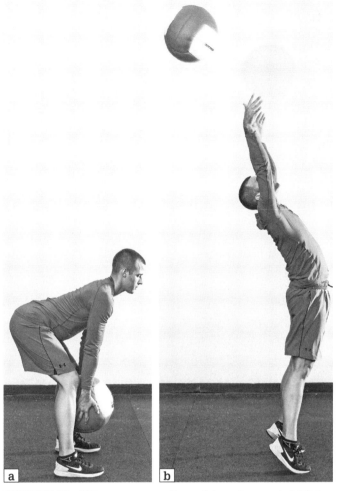

FIGURE 5.16   MB reverse scoop throw: *(a)* quarter squat; *(b)* throw.

Stability Balls

Stability balls (SB) have been used as an exercise tool since the late 1980s. They have undergone a significant evolution in design and materials. When they first entered the strength and conditioning world, they were often used to provide an unstable training environment. As functional training evolved, we realized that the overuse of balance and unstable training was not helpful for the high power transfer of sport. This realization, along with a few unfortunate accidents, has forced the industry to reevaluate the use of the stability balls as an unstable support surface for heavy training (e.g., heavy bench pressing and squatting on the ball). We prefer to use the stability ball for three main purposes:

1. To support dynamic positions in a stationary environment (e.g., single-leg lateral wall slides)

2. To support what could be a dangerous position in a safe environment (e.g., extension and flexion of the spine)

3. To provide a rolling surface that facilitates movement and natural instability

This section offers a selection of exercises in each of these three categories.

SB Single-Leg Lateral Wall Slide

Details and Benefits

- Progression from other single-leg exercises
- One of the most effective exercises to develop lateral changes of direction without any wear and tear on the ankle and knee joints, making it great for field and court athletes

Starting Position

- Stand with a wall to the right of you.
- Place a stability ball between your armpit and the wall, with the right arm resting on the ball and the hand placed on the wall for balance.
- Walk approximately 2 feet (.5 m) to the left to create a right lean against the ball and lift the right foot (inside foot), balancing on the left foot (outside foot) (figure 5.17a).

Movement

- Perform mini squats on the left leg as you lean against the ball and use your right arm on the ball and right hand on the wall for balance (figure 5.17b).
- Place the right foot next to the left and lift the left foot off the ground.
- Perform mini squats with your left leg.
- Perform on the other side.

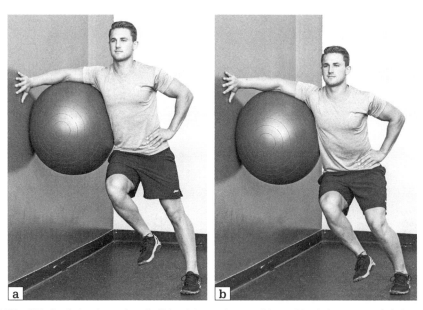

FIGURE 5.17 SB single-leg lateral wall slide: *(a)* starting position; *(b)* mini squat on left leg.

SB Hands-on-Ball Push-Up

Details and Benefits

- Natural progression from all push-up and plank progressions
- Go-to progression to develop core and shoulder stabilization if winging scapulae and a weak core are observed on a regular push-up

Starting Position

- Assume a plank position with your hands on the stability ball, making sure the hands are on the outer sides of the ball, fingers pointing toward the ground (figure 5.18a).
- The core should be tight and the knees should be extended, with weight on the balls of feet and feet shoulder-width apart.

Movement

- Flex the elbows to lower the chest until it is a few inches from the ball (figure 5.18b).
- Finish by extending the arms to return to plank position.
- To decrease the intensity of this exercise, place the ball on a higher surface or secure it between the floor and the wall.

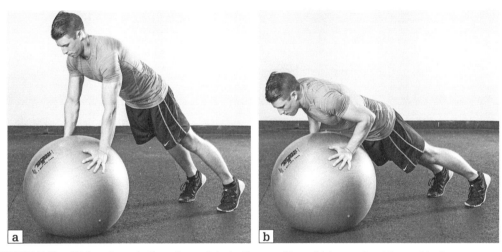

FIGURE 5.18   SB hands-on-ball push-up: *(a)* starting position; *(b)* lower chest toward ball.

SB Knee Tuck (Double Leg to Single Leg)

Details and Benefits

- This exercise is an intermediate progression from any core flexion exercise and push-ups.
- It's a great anterior core exercise that also requires strong shoulder stabilization, making it popular with athletes who require tucking and shoulder stability, such as gymnasts, divers, and combat athletes.
- It's described as a two-leg exercise here, but the goal is to perform it on a single leg as soon as multiple sets of 15 repetitions can be performed with two legs.

Starting Position

- Assume a push-up position with the hands on the ground and the stability ball under the middle to lower thighs (figure 5.19a).
- Keep the core tight and avoid hyperextending the spine.

Movement

- Stabilizing the movement with the hands, keep the core tight and flex at the hips and knees, tucking the knees in toward the chest.
- Continue hip and knee flexion until the hips and knees are flexed 90 degrees and knees are on top of the stability ball (figure 5.19b). For additional flexibility, the tuck can be tighter.
- Extend the body back to the starting position.
- Repeat the tucking motion.

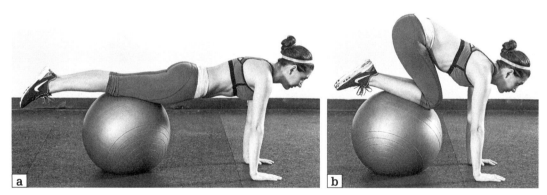

FIGURE 5.19 SB knee tuck (double leg): *(a)* starting position; *(b)* tuck.

SB Rollout

Details and Benefits
- Natural progression from planks, push-ups, and anterior core work
- Versatile progression to lengthen and strengthen the anterior core, as well as strengthen the shoulder joint, making it popular with swimmers, throwing athletes, and combat athletes

Starting Position
- My favorite rollout progression is performed on a wall because it offers the safest application while delivering excellent intensity. However, you can attempt more advanced progressions with the ball on the ground with varying arm positions (e.g., from hand or from elbows).
- Hold a stability ball in front of you and against a wall, your arms extended and palms on the ball as if you were in a plank position, balancing between the balls of your feet and the ball (figure 5.20a).
- To increase the intensity of the rollout, walk your feet away from the wall and stand on the balls of your feet.

Movement
- Keeping your body stiff, allow your shoulders to open, and roll your hands and forearms over the ball until your body is fully extended.
- In the extended position you should be on the balls of your feet with the ball closer to your shoulders (figure 5.20b).
- Once fully extended, use your pulling muscles to pull your arms back, rolling them over the ball to the starting plank position.

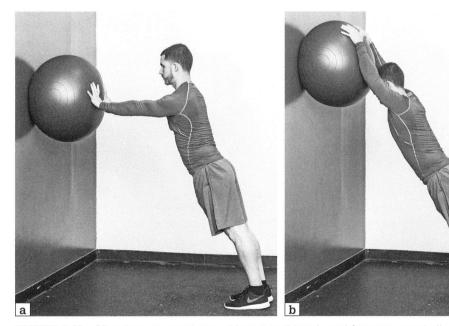

FIGURE 5.20 SB rollout: *(a)* starting position; *(b)* roll hands and forearms over ball.

SB Bridge (Double Leg to Single Leg)

Details and Benefits

- This is one of the most basic and effective progressions for simultaneously strengthening the posterior core and stretching the anterior core.
- It's essential for any athlete who runs, and it's our most common hamstring rehabilitator.
- It's described as a two-leg exercise here, but the goal is to perform it on a single leg as soon as multiple sets of 15 repetitions can be performed with two legs.

Starting Position

- Lie on your back with arms out about 45 degrees and palms down.
- Place the stability ball under the calves (easier) or the ankles (harder) while keeping the knees and ankles together.
- Keeping the knees slightly bent, lift the hips toward the ceiling until a bridge forms between the shoulders on the ground and the legs on the ball (figure 5.21a).

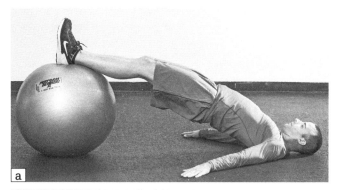

Movement

- Lower the hips short of touching the ground (figure 5.21b) and return to the bridge position.
- Repeat.

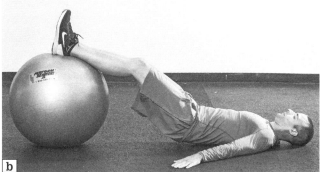

FIGURE 5.21 SB bridge (double leg): (a) starting position; (b) lower the hips.

SB Hip Lift (Double Leg to Single Leg)

The SB hip lift is a basic to intermediate progression that follows the SB bridge. It simultaneously strengthens the posterior core and stretches the anterior core while involving the calves. It is an outstanding progression to strengthen the hamstrings and improve stride length and running speed. Like the SB bridge, this exercise is described as a two-leg exercise here, but the goal is to perform it on a single leg as soon as multiple sets of 15 repetitions can be performed with two legs.

The starting position is similar to the SB bridge, but the foot position is different. Lie on your back with arms out about 45 degrees and palms down. Place the stability ball under the balls of the feet while keeping the knees and ankles together. Bring the hips toward the ceiling until a bridge forms between the shoulders on the ground and the feet on the ball (figure 5.22a). Lower the hips short of touching the ground (figure 5.22b) and repeat the bridging motion.

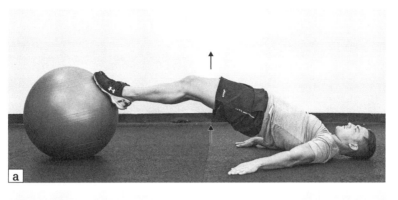

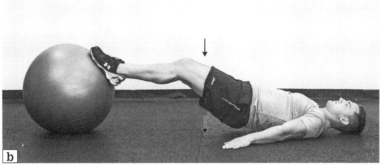

FIGURE 5.22 SB hip lift (double leg): *(a)* bridge; *(b)* lower hips.

SB Leg Curl (Double Leg to Single Leg)

Details and Benefits

- This is a basic hamstring rehabilitation exercise and an effective way to develop the hamstrings as knee flexors.
- It's essential for any athlete who runs or combat athletes who use the guard position from their backs.
- It's described as a two-leg exercise here, but the goal is to perform it on a single leg as soon as multiple sets of 15 repetitions can be performed with two legs.

Starting Position

- Lie on your back with arms out about 45 degrees and palms down.
- Place the stability ball between the calves (easier) or the ankles (harder) while keeping the knees and ankles together.
- Bring the hips toward the ceiling until a bridge forms between the shoulders on the ground and the feet on the ball (figure 5.23a).
- Keep the hips elevated during the entire movement.

Movement

- Flex the knees and roll the feet over the ball and back toward the glutes (figure 5.23b).
- Extend the legs until the knees are almost fully extended to return to starting position.
- Repeat the knee flexion movement while keeping the hips elevated.

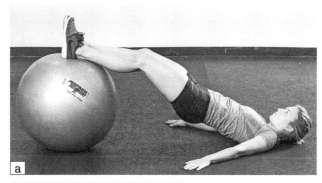

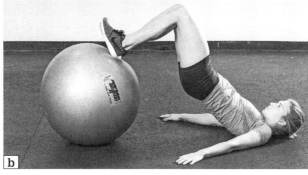

FIGURE 5.23 SB leg curl (double leg): *(a)* starting position; *(b)* flex the knees.

SB Hyperextension

Details and Benefits

- Basic progression that can assist all squatting, deadlift, and reaching lunge variations
- Outstanding progression to strengthen the middle to upper paraspinal muscles used in flexed athletic positions as well as lifting in combat sports

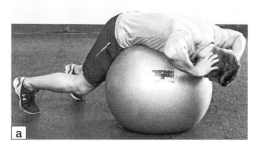

Starting Position

- Kneel on both knees and place a stability ball under the abdominal area.
- While balancing on the ball and the balls of your feet, extend the legs (keeping the knees slightly bent) to lift the knees off the ground.
- Place your hands by the sides of your head (i.e., cupping the ears) and balance on the ball and the balls of the feet.

Movement

- Curl the core around the ball (figure 5.24a), and then extend the spine as much as you can without pain or pressure in the lower back (figure 5.24b).
- Curl the core around the ball and repeat the extension movement.

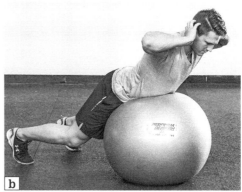

FIGURE 5.24 SB hyperextension: *(a)* curl core around ball; *(b)* extend spine.

SB Reverse Hyperextension

Details and Benefits

- Basic progression to deadlift and squatting progressions
- Perfect complement to SB hyperextension, working the lower portion of the paraspinal muscles, glutes, and hamstrings

Starting Position

- Kneel on both knees and place a stability ball under the abdominal region.
- Roll over the ball until both forearms are flat on the ground, and extend the legs and hips completely, keeping the knees and feet together (figure 5.25a).

Movement

- Balancing on both forearms and the ball, slowly flex at the hips until your feet almost touch the ground (figure 5.25b).
- Slowly extend the hips until your body is perfectly straight again, pausing slightly at the top of the movement.
- Keep your legs straight and stiff throughout the entire movement.

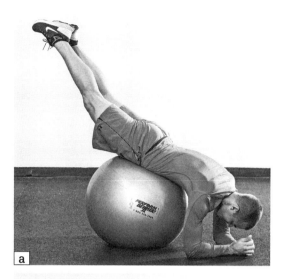

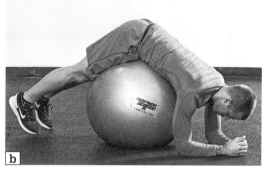

FIGURE 5.25 SB reverse hyperextension: *(a)* starting position; *(b)* flex at hips to lower feet toward ground.

SB Log Roll

Details and Benefits

- Intermediate progression that follows the SB knee tuck and the T push-up (chapter 4); regression to the SB skier
- Extended position reduces stability demands but maintains a high range of motion at the thoracic spine
- Premier exercise for golfers and combat athletes who require excellent upper-spine (i.e. thoracic spine) mobility.

Starting Position

- Assume a push-up position with the hands on the ground and the stability ball under the thighs.
- Maintain eye contact with the ground at all times.
- Keep the core tight and avoid hyperextending the spine.

Movement

- Stabilizing the movement with the hands, rotate your hips to the right so that the outside of the right thigh rests on top of the ball (figure 5.26a).
- Turn your hips to the left until the outside of the left thigh rests on top of the ball (figure 5.26b).
- For more spinal rotation, keep your arms straight during the movement. For less spinal rotation, allows the elbows to flex during the rotation.
- Repeat the rotational motion to both sides.

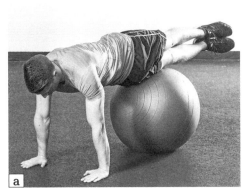

FIGURE 5.26 SB log roll: (a) rotate hips to the left; (b) rotate hips to the right.

SB Skier

Details and Benefits

- Intermediate to advanced progression that follows the SB log roll, SB knee tuck, push-up, and plank
- Great rotational core exercise that also requires strong shoulder stabilization, making it popular with skiers, surfers, combat athletes, and golfers

Starting Position

- Assume a push-up position with the hands on the ground and the stability ball under the thighs.
- Tuck the knees in toward the chest until the hips and knees are flexed 90 degrees and knees are on top of the ball (figure 5.27a).

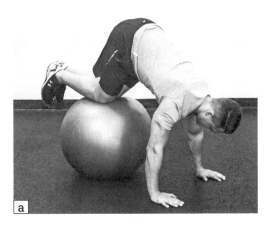

Movement

- Stabilizing the movement with the hands, rotate your hips to the right so that the outside of the left thigh rests on top of the ball (figure 5.27b).
- For more spinal rotation, keep your arms straight during the movement. For less spinal rotation, allow the elbows to flex during the rotation.
- Repeat the skiing motion to both sides.

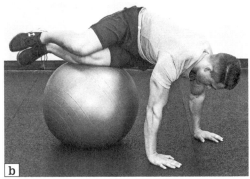

FIGURE 5.27 SB skier: (a) starting position; (b) rotate hips to the right.

Toys

No functional training book would be complete without showcasing some of the more popular functional toys. I have chosen five of the most popular pieces of equipment used for sport stability, agility, quickness, and power. This equipment is also easy to get and inexpensive, and most pieces travel easily. The exercises in this section are simple ones that produce excellent results, and they integrate well with the exercise programming in this book.

Note: Always make sure to read and follow all manufacturer recommendations, warnings, and instructions before using the equipment for any exercise. If you have any questions or doubts on how to use this equipment, consult a certified fitness professional well versed in functional speed, agility, and quickness training.

Vibration Blade Throw

Details and Benefits

- A vibration blade or stick is a great piece of equipment that can transmit vibration to any part of the body. The two main models are the Flexi-Bar (provides vibration along all planes of motion like a fishing rod does) and the Bodyblade (provides vibration along one plane of motion like a bow does). The Bodyblade is easier to control, whereas the Flexi-Bar offer much more of a challenge.

- The vibratory stimulus improves the stabilization of the shoulders and to a lesser degree the spine and hips.

- This exercise is excellent for athletes who use a throwing motion.

Starting Position

- Assume a split stance.

- The distance between your feet should be the same as the distance from the top of your hips to the floor.

- The feet should be hip-width apart, with the left foot to the front, both knees slightly bent in an athletic position, and the right heel off the ground.

Movement

- Keeping the core tight, hold the vibration blade in the right hand and start oscillating it up and down without using a strong grip. The movement should be short (a few inches), it should be easy, and it should come from the shoulder. The oscillation of the blade should not move (i.e., shake) the core or hips.

- While oscillating the vibration blade, perform a throwing motion with the arm (figure 5.28). Repeat to complete the recommended number of repetitions.

- Change your stance and perform with the left arm.

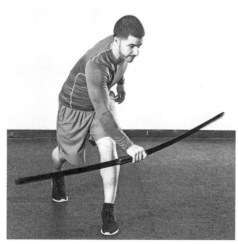

FIGURE 5.28 Vibration blade throw.

Vibration Blade 12 O'Clock Oscillation

Details and Benefits
- Sends vibratory stimulus to the core of the body to activate the muscles that create core stiffness
- Fantastic finesse exercise to activate the core muscles during rehab or light training, making it perfect to prepare an athlete for intense rotational exercise
- Excellent at improving muscle control during batting and golf swings

Starting Position
- Stand with feet shoulder-width apart and knees slightly bent.
- Hold the vibration blade vertically in both hands with a hand-over-hand grip.

Movement
- Keep the entire body tight and start oscillating the vibration blade side to side without using a strong grip (figure 5.29).
- The oscillation should be short (a few inches), easy, come from the shoulders, and transmit to a stiff core.
- The oscillation of the bar should not move (i.e., shake) the core or hips.

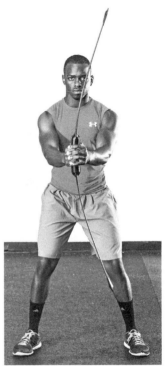

FIGURE 5.29 Vibration blade 12 o'clock oscillation.

Agility Ladder Split Step

Details and Benefits
- This is the most popular piece of court or field equipment for developing agility and foot speed.
- It has elements of hopscotch and rope skipping along with lateral and reactive components.
- It's a simple exercise used to develop ankle stability and improve the components of deceleration and lateral changes in direction.
- It's excellent for field and court athletes, such as soccer, tennis, and basketball players.
- Use a full ladder (10 yd [9 m]) to learn the movement. Use a half ladder (5 yd [5 m]) to develop speed once the movement is mastered.

Starting Position
- Stand at the end of the ladder.
- Feet are shoulder-width apart and knees are slightly bent.

Movement
- Jump with both feet into the first box of the ladder (figure 5.30).
- Jump to the outside of the next rung, straddling the ladder, and immediately into the next box with both feet.

- Repeat the in-and-out pattern through the entire ladder, jumping into every box.
- Stay on the balls of the feet during the exercise.
- Work on developing a steady rhythm before increasing speed.

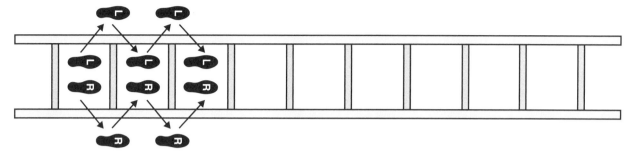

FIGURE 5.30   Agility ladder split step.

Agility Ladder Lateral Rotational Jump

Details and Benefits
- This is an excellent progression from the agility ladder split step and a complement to the BP rotation.
- It improves the short shuffling and rotational jumping necessary in sports with complex foot movements, such as boxing and soccer.
- Use a full ladder (10 yd [9 m]) to learn the movement. Use a half ladder (5 yd [5 m]) to develop speed once the movement is mastered.

Starting Position
- Stand at the end of the ladder with the ladder in front and to the right of you. Place the right foot inside of the first box and the left outside the ladder to the left of the first box.
- Feet are shoulder-width apart and knees are slightly bent.

Movement
- Jump to the right, rotating your hips 90 degrees to the right while simultaneously placing your left foot in the first box and right foot outside the second box (figure 5.31).
- As soon as you land, jump to the right, rotating your hips 90 degrees to the left while simultaneously placing your right foot in the second box and left foot outside the first box.
- As you move to the right on the ladder, the right foot leads and the left foot always follows the placement of the right foot.
- Repeat the sequence down the ladder. When you get to the end of the ladder, come back, repeating the same sequence to the left.
- As you move to the left on the ladder, the left foot leads and the right foot follows the placement of the left foot.

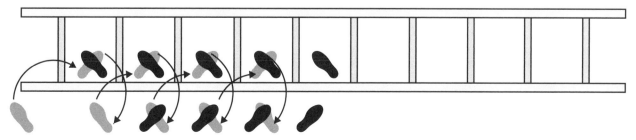

FIGURE 5.31   Agility ladder lateral rotational jump.

Low-Hurdle Run

Details and Benefits

- Several models and materials are available. Low hurdles are about 6 to 8 inches (15-20 cm) high and are used to cue knee lifting or jumping. Most drills can use 6 to 10 hurdles.

- This exercise is excellent for progressing from the warm-up and for supplementing running and biomotor skills.

- It improves the hip flexion power and knee lift needed during the acceleration phase of running.

Starting Position

- Place 6 to 10 hurdles 20 to 24 inches (51-61 cm) apart, depending on the athlete's size and ability and the speed of the drill.

- Stand about 2 feet (61 cm) in front of the first hurdle.

Movement

- Run over each hurdle (figure 5.32), placing the left foot between the first and second hurdles, placing the right foot between the second and third hurdles, and repeating the sequence through the entire line of hurdles.

- Stay on the balls of your plant foot while concentrating on high knee lift and keeping the foot and toes up on the opposite leg.

- Keep your posture upright and straight and your elbows at 90 degrees. Rotate your arms at the shoulders, not the elbows.

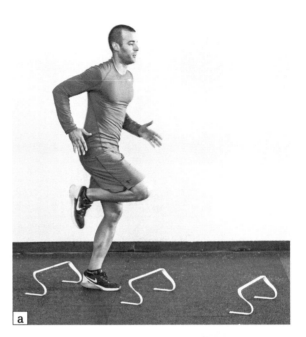

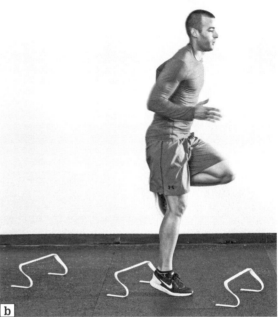

FIGURE 5.32 Low-hurdle run: *(a)* left foot between first and second hurdles; *(b)* right foot between second and third hurdles.

Low-Hurdle Diagonal Jump

Details and Benefits

- Excellent progression to intensify low-amplitude jumping progressions
- Improves the ankle stability and stiffness necessary for reactive jumping and running

Starting Position

- Place 6 to 10 hurdles in a zigzag pattern at 90 degrees to each other.
- Stand outside the first hurdle with feet close together and knees slightly bent.

Movement

- Jump across each hurdle diagonally, always facing the end of the hurdle line (figure 5.33).

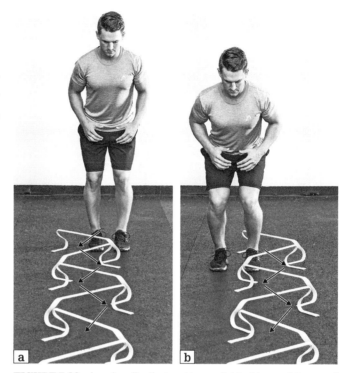

FIGURE 5.33 Low-hurdle diagonal jump: *(a)* first jump; *(b)* second jump.

- Stay on the balls of the feet and keep the feet and knees together. Keep the elbows bent 90 degrees and relaxed.

Crooked Stick Hexagon Drill

Details and Benefits

- The crooked stick is a cheap, diverse, easy-to-use tool that provides many patterns for agility drills.
- The crooked stick hexagon drill is an excellent progression that has been long used in the assessment and development of agility.
- It improves and evaluates agility used in field and court sports, such as tennis and soccer.

Starting Position

- Set up the crooked stick in a hexagon pattern.
- Stand in the middle of the hexagon with feet close together and knees slightly bent.

Movement

- Jump with both feet to the top of the hexagon and then back to the middle (figure 5.34).

- Always facing the top of the hexagon, continue jumping clockwise to each side of the hexagon, always returning to the middle until the entire hexagon is complete.
- Perform three round trips clockwise, rest, and then three round trips counterclockwise. This equals one set.
- Time how long it takes to complete each of the three round trip in each direction. You will find out which direction is your weakest and how training improves your movement symmetry.

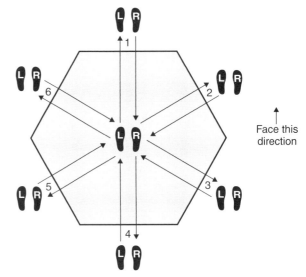

FIGURE 5.34   Crooked stick hexagon drill.

- Keep your posture upright and elbows at 90 degrees. Always face the front of the hexagon.

Crooked Stick Cross-Rotational Jump Drill

Details and Benefits

- Excellent progression from and supplement to the agility ladder lateral rotation jump
- Improves the ability to reposition the feet in short quarters as used in combat and court sports, such as judo and basketball

Starting Position

- Set up the crooked stick in a cross pattern.
- Stand with a segment between your legs and the intersection and the other three segments of the stick in front of you.
- Stand with your feet shoulder-width apart and knees slightly bent.

Movement

- Jump with both feet to the right as you rotate left, landing on the right perpendicular segment (figure 5.35).
- Jump again with both feet to the right as you rotate left, landing on the right perpendicular segment (now you are facing opposite where you started).
- Perform two more jumps until you land in the starting position. Repeat counterclockwise.

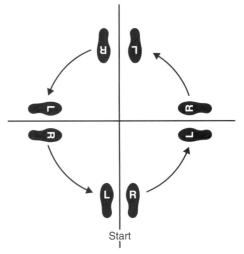

FIGURE 5.35   Crooked stick cross-rotational jump drill.

Ropes Alternating Up and Down

Details and Benefits

- Ropes are cheap, diverse, and easy-to-use tools that provide excellent core and upper-body stability and endurance.
- Ropes can be 40 to 60 feet (12-15 m) long and 1.5 to 2 inches (4-5 cm) in diameter.
- Ropes alternating up and down is an advanced progression from the vibration blade throw and the DB horizontal fly rotation.
- The exercise improves shoulder stability and endurance along with enhancing core stability, making it popular for throwers and combat athletes, such as pitchers and wrestlers.

Starting Position

- Wrap the rope around a sturdy structure so the two halves of the ropes match in length.
- Stand with the ropes stretched out and in your hands.
- Take a step toward the anchor point so that you create slack in the rope.
- Hold one end of the rope in each hand, place your feet shoulder-width apart, and keep your knees slightly bent.

Movement

- Keeping your core tight, move the right hand up and the left hand down simultaneously, creating an undulating wave with each rope that is as high as your shoulder line (figure 5.36).
- Try to keep your hips and core from moving. Maintain a stiff core.
- Perform for time or repetitions as specified.

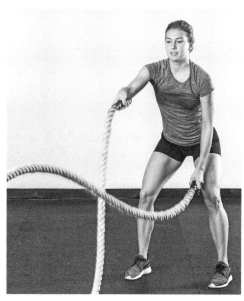

FIGURE 5.36   Ropes alternating up and down.

Rope Circles (Clockwise and Counterclockwise)

Details and Benefits

- This is a progression from and supplement to the vibration blade throw and the DB horizontal fly rotation.
- It improves shoulder stability, specifically internal and external rotation, and it enhances core stability.
- This is a great exercise for improving the throwing motion, such as serving in tennis, spiking in volleyball, and throwing in baseball.

Starting Position

- Wrap the rope around a sturdy structure so the two halves of the ropes match in length.
- Stand with the ropes stretched out and in your hands.
- Take a step toward the anchor point so that you create slack in the rope.
- Hold one end of the rope in each hand, place your feet shoulder-width apart, and keep your knees slightly bent.

Movement

- Simultaneously make outward circles with each hand (figure 5.37), creating circles with each rope that are as high as your shoulder line.
- The left hand moves counterclockwise while the right hand moves clockwise.
- Try to keep your hips and core from moving. Maintain a stiff core.
- Perform for time or repetitions as specified.

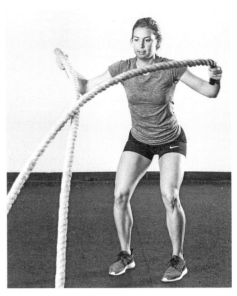

FIGURE 5.37 Rope circles (clockwise and counterclockwise).

Lateral Slide

Details and Benefits

- A slide is a board with a slippery surface that is used with special "booties" to simulate skating motions. It makes a great piece of equipment to improve lateral changes of directions with minimal impact.
- The lateral slide is a great movement for lateral changes in direction and high-speed acceleration.
- It improves lower-body strength and hip stability, specifically internal and external rotation of the hip while extending the leg.
- It's great for improving cutting ability in field and court athletes and for athletes involved in skating.
- It can be loaded by using a vest or attaching a light band to the waist of the athlete and providing a lateral resistance.
- The most common length for sliding is 6 to 8 feet (1.8-2.4 m), although 4- or 5-foot (1-1.5 m) lengths can be used to learn the movement.
- Learn the movement before attempting the exercise to avoid pulled muscles on the insides of the legs.

Starting Position

- Place the slide on a nonslip surface and put the booties (shoe covers) suggested by the manufacturer over your shoes. The booties protect the slide and allow for a smooth glide over the surface.

- Stand on the left end of the slide with the outside of the left foot contacting the left-side end board.
- Bend your knees and hips and get in an athletic position, as if you are getting ready to change lateral directions (figure 5.38a).

Movement

- Push hard off the end board with the left foot while staying low and in the athletic position.
- Glide across the slide board in a low, wide stance until your right foot makes contact with the right end board (figure 5.38b).
- Absorb the impact by bending the right leg. Immediately push off and slide to the left.
- Continue the side-to-side skating motion while keeping a low, wide stance.

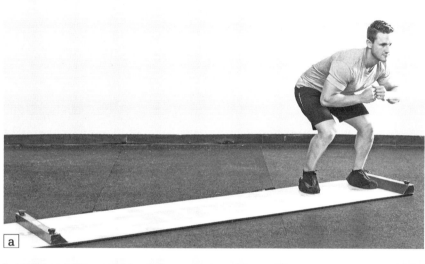

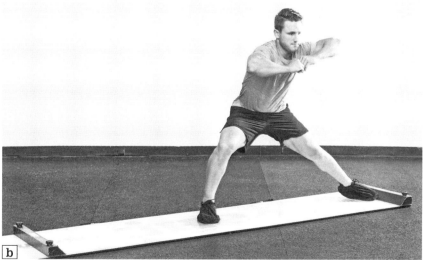

FIGURE 5.38 Lateral slide: *(a)* starting position; *(b)* slide.

Slide Running

Details and Benefits

- Great movement for the knee lift needed in running as well as kicking and kneeing in combat sports
- Improves core lower-body strength, specifically the hip flexor complex
- Popular with sprinters and combat athletes

Starting Position

- Place the slide on a nonslip surface and put the booties (shoe covers) suggested by the manufacturer over your shoes. The booties protect the slide and allow for a smooth glide over the surface.
- Get into a plank position with your hands on the floor just outside the end board and your feet in the middle of the slide.
- Flex the right hip and knee about 90 degrees to slide the right foot toward your chest while keeping the left leg extended (figure 5.39a).
- Keep the core and shoulders stable and tight throughout the movement.

Movement

- Explosively extend the right leg as you flex the left hip and knee to bring the left foot toward your chest (figure 5.39b).
- Continue the running motion for the repetitions or time indicated while keeping the shoulders and core tight.

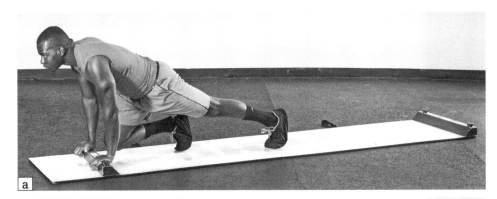

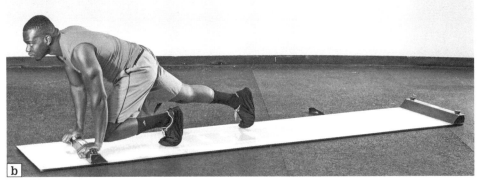

FIGURE 5.39 Slide running: *(a)* starting position; *(b)* extend right leg and flex left hip and knee.

Traditional Strength Exercises

Many fitness experts do not consider traditional training with free weights and resistance training machines to be functional training. However, if fast hypertrophy is desired, traditional weight training can certainly provide it. Therefore, many athletes looking for additional muscle mass and function will need a system that seamlessly combines traditional training and functional training. To help create such a system, I have provided some common traditional exercises that will add strength and size to any athlete who needs them. In the programming part of the book, I cover how to combine traditional bodybuilding exercises and functional training. Unlike the more comprehensive descriptions of the functional exercises, this section provides a brief description and pictures depicting the starting and movement positions.

I am providing only a few examples of traditional exercises, and many variations exist. For example, a barbell exercise such as the barbell squat can be done with dumbbells with equal effectiveness. The same goes for a dumbbell exercise such as the dumbbell bent-over row; a barbell version can easily take its place. Resistance training machines and free weights can be used interchangeably. For example, a barbell flat bench press can be substituted for a chest press machine. Substituting like-for-like exercises can make it much easier to adapt a program to meet your needs.

Machine Leg Press

The leg press is a traditional strength exercise that targets the entire lower body.

Starting Position

- Sit in the leg press.
- Put your feet in the middle of the foot-plate, feet facing forward and shoulder-width apart.

Movement

- Extend your legs to lift the weight and unlock the safety mechanism (figure 5.40a).
- Flex the knees and lower the weight as far as you can without lifting the hips off the seat or rounding the lower back (figure 5.40b).
- Extend the legs to full extension and repeat the pressing movement.
- Make sure the lower back is always firmly against the backrest and the glutes remain on the seat through the entire movement.

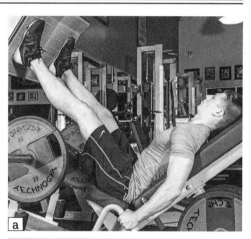

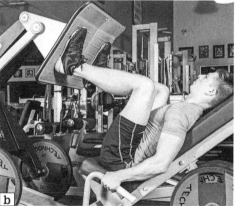

FIGURE 5.40 Machine leg press: *(a)* Extend legs; *(b)* lower weight.

Barbell Squat

The barbell squat is known as the king of all lifts due to its impact on the whole body, especially the core and legs.

Starting Position

- Set up a rack with the barbell just below shoulder-height and the safety racks about 1 to 2 inches (3-5 cm) below your expected squatting level.
- Hold the bar symmetrically with the hands well outside shoulder-width apart.
- Walk under the bar and let it rest on the fleshy part of the trapezius muscles, just below the neck.

Movement

- Stand up with the weight and feel the balance.
- Step back a couple of steps and stand with your feet shoulder-width apart while remaining over the safety racks (figure 5.41a).
- Keeping the core tight and chest up, hinge at the hips and flex the knees to lower the weight (figure 5.41b).
- When you get to the desired squat depth, stand up to complete the repetition.

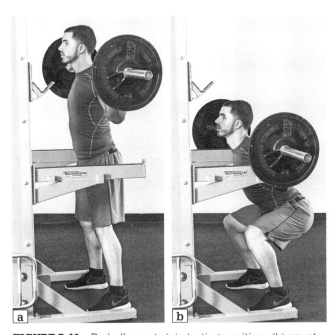

FIGURE 5.41 Barbell squat: *(a)* starting position; *(b)* squat.

Barbell Deadlift

The barbell deadlift is a core strength lift that targets the lower back, glutes, and hamstrings. There are numerous deadlift variations. This is the Olympic lifting version used with most of our athletes.

Starting Position

- Place a barbell on the ground. Approach the bar until it contacts the shins while the feet are hip-width apart.
- Keeping your back straight and core braced, flex the knees and hips to lower the body and grip the bar outside hip-width apart.

Movement

- Once you grip the bar, continue bracing the core and drive with the legs to initiate the lift (figure 5.42a).
- As the bar comes up along the shins, the legs extend to clear the bar past the knees.
- Once the bar clears the knees, finish the lift with hip extension until your body is fully extended and upright (figure 5.42b).
- Reverse the movement to bring the bar back to the ground.

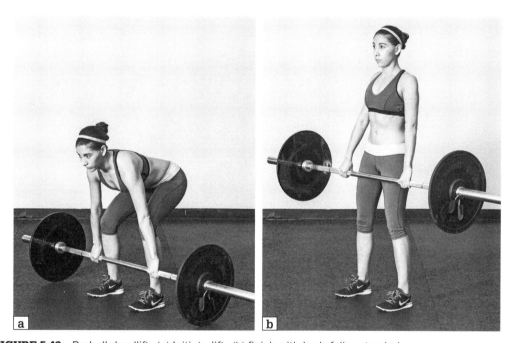

FIGURE 5.42 Barbell deadlift: (a) Initiate lift; (b) finish with body fully extended.

45-Degree Back Extension

The 45-degree back extension is excellent for the entire posterior chain.

Starting Position

- Position rollers or pads well below the hip line so that the hips can freely hinge.
- Place your thighs on the thigh pads and put your feet on the platform, hooking the heels under the leg pads.
- Keep the feet facing forward to target the hamstrings, or point the feet outward to focus more on the glutes.
- Place your hands across your chest or to the sides of your head. For additional resistance, you may hold a medicine ball or weight plate at your chest.
- Maintain a slight bend in the knees throughout the movement to avoid hyperextending the knees and to better engage the hamstrings.

Movement

- Keeping your chest up, back straight, and knees slightly bent, hinge at the hips to lower the upper body (figure 5.43a).
- Go as low as you can without bending the spine.
- At the bottom of the hip flexion, squeeze your glutes and hamstrings to fully extend the body until it is perfectly straight (figure 5.43b).

Single-Leg 45-Degree Back Extension

You can increase the intensity of this exercise by progressing to the single-leg variation (figure 5.44).

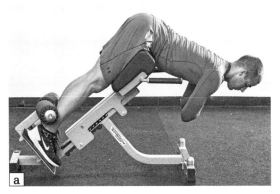

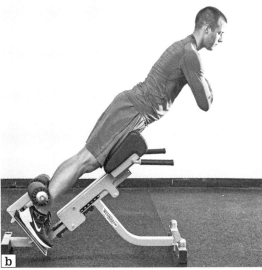

FIGURE 5.43 45-degree back extension: *(a)* Lower the upper body; *(b)* extend the body.

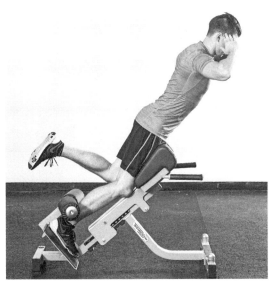

FIGURE 5.44 Single-leg 45-degree back extension.

Barbell Flat Bench Press

The barbell flat bench press is the most common exercise used to build and strengthen the upper body, primarily the chest, anterior shoulders, and triceps.

Starting Position

- Lie on a flat bench with your feet flat on the ground and your back and head supported by the bench at all times.
- Grip the bar with a prone grip (palms down), hands just outside shoulder-width apart.
- Remove the barbell from the rack, holding the bar with straight arms vertically in line with the shoulder joints (figure 5.45a).

Movement

- Lower the bar to the middle of the chest, keeping the elbows aligned under the bar at all times (figure 5.45b).
- When the bar is at its lowest point, press it back to the starting position.

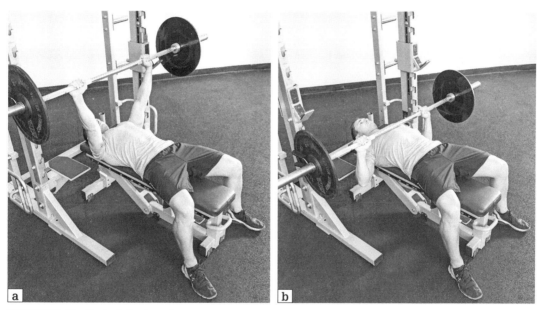

FIGURE 5.45 Barbell flat bench press: (a) starting position; (b) lower bar.

Barbell Incline Bench Press

The barbell incline bench press is a popular upper-body exercise that places a greater emphasis on the shoulders and upper fibers of the chest while also working the triceps.

Starting Position

- Use a dedicated incline bench or set up a rack and adjustable bench at 30 to 45 degrees.
- Lie on the incline bench with your feet flat on the ground and with your back and head supported by the bench at all times.
- Grip the bar with a prone grip, hands just outside shoulder-width apart.
- Remove the barbell from the rack, holding the bar with straight arms vertically in line with the shoulder joints (figure 5.46a).

Movement

- Lower the bar to midchest, keeping the elbows aligned under the bar at all times (figure 5.46b).
- When the bar is at its lowest point, press it back to the starting position.

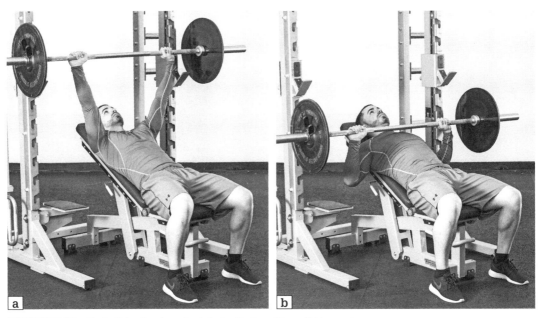

FIGURE 5.46 Barbell incline bench: *(a)* starting position; *(b)* lower bar.

Barbell Overhead Press

The barbell overhead press strengthens the shoulders and upper arms, primarily the deltoids, trapezius, and triceps. This exercise can be performed on a dedicated shoulder press bench or while standing and using a weight rack. The standing version is presented here.

Starting Position

- Set up a rack with the bar just under shoulder-height.
- Make sure to use safety racks set at chest-height in case of an emergency.
- Grip the bar with a prone grip, hands just outside shoulder-width apart.

Movement

- Lift the bar, stabilize it at the clavicle (collarbone), and walk back a couple of steps while still staying in the safety rack area (figure 5.47a).
- Press the bar overhead until the arms are locked and the weight is vertically aligned with the head, shoulders, hips, knees, and ankles (figure 5.47b).
- Lower the bar to the starting position.

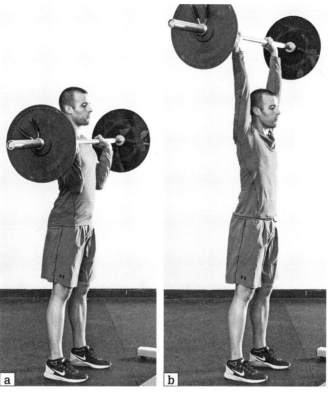

FIGURE 5.47 Barbell overhead press: *(a)* starting position; *(b)* press bar overhead.

Pull-Down

The pull-down is a traditional strength exercise that targets the muscles of the back, primarily the latissimus dorsi, as well as the biceps and forearms. This exercise can be done with a pin-loaded machine or a cable with a bar at the end. The pin-loaded machine version is described here.

Starting Position

- Set up the seat height so that you can sit down and reach the bar overhead.
- Sit down on the seat and grab the handles.
- Grip the bar in a prone grip, hands just outside shoulder-width apart.
- Set and stabilize the shoulder blades by bringing them down and back.
- Look straight ahead while slightly arching the spine to stabilize the core.

Movement

- Keep the core tight and slowly pull the handles close to clavicle (collarbone) level, right above the chest (figure 5.48a).
- Once the handles reach the lowest position, slowly allow them to return to the starting position (figure 5.48b).

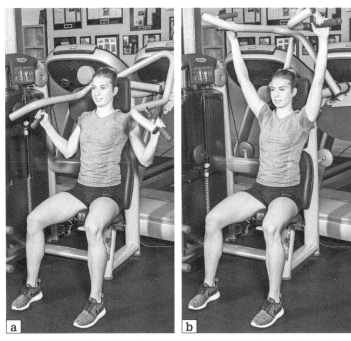

FIGURE 5.48 Pull-down: *(a)* Pull the handles down; *(b)* slowly return the handles to the up position.

Seated Row

The seated row is a pulling exercise that targets the back and biceps. This exercise can be done with a pin-loaded machine or a cable with a handle or bar at the end. The pin-loaded version is described here.

Starting Position

- Sit on the seat with the feet flat on the floor or on a footplate if present. The knees should be bent, back is upright, and the chest is in contact with the chest pad.
- Reach forward to hold the handles. The arms should be straight.
- Keep the shoulders back on this exercise, and maintain a straight line between the hand and wrist (figure 5.49a).

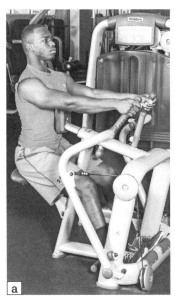
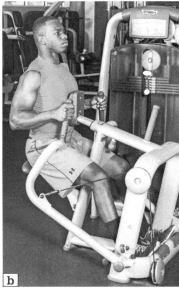

FIGURE 5.49 Seated cable row: *(a)* starting position; *(b)* row.

Movement

- Keeping the chest against the chest pad, perform a rowing motion (figure 5.49b), bending the elbows (which should travel directly backward) until the hands are just in front of the stomach.
- Slowly return toward the starting position and stop once the elbows are almost straight before repeating the exercise.

Dumbbell Bent-Over Row

The dumbbell bent-over row is a traditional back exercise that also targets the biceps and forearms. Several foot positions and stabilizing methods can be used for this exercise. The bench-stabilized parallel-stance version is described here.

Starting Position

- Stand 2 to 3 feet (.5-1 m) away from a bench or other low, stable structure.
- Place a dumbbell between you and the bench.
- Set your feet shoulder-width apart.
- Place your left hand on the bench, slightly flexing both knees and stabilizing your core.
- Keep your core and shoulders tight and parallel to the ground at all times.

Movement

- Take hold of the dumbbell with the right hand (figure 5.50a).
- Making sure your back is straight and set, row the dumbbell to the side of your ribcage (figure 5.50b). The only movement should come from the right shoulder and arm.
- Once the dumbbell reaches the body, slowly lower it until the right arm is fully extended.
- Repeat the rowing motion and perform on both sides of the body.

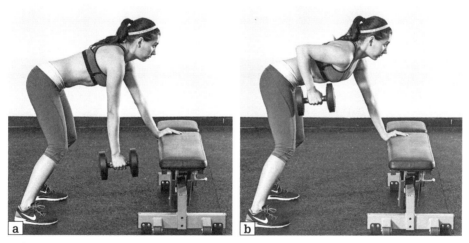

FIGURE 5.50 Dumbbell bent-over row: *(a)* starting position; *(b)* row.

Barbell Upright Row

The barbell upright row is an upper-body pulling exercise that strengthens the muscles of the upper back and the lateral and rear aspects of the shoulders. This exercise can be performed with dumbbells, a cable and bar, or a barbell.

Starting Position

- Hold a barbell with a prone grip, hands slightly outside hip-width apart.
- The feet should be hip-width apart, knees slightly bent.
- The hips are slightly flexed and the core of the body is straight and tight throughout the movement.
- Align the body vertically so there is a line through the shoulders, hips, knees, and ankles (figure 5.51a).

Movement

- Pull the barbell straight up until it is at the bottom of the chest and the elbows are horizontally in line with the shoulders (figure 5.51b).
- Slowly lower the weight until the arms are straight.
- Repeat the upright row.

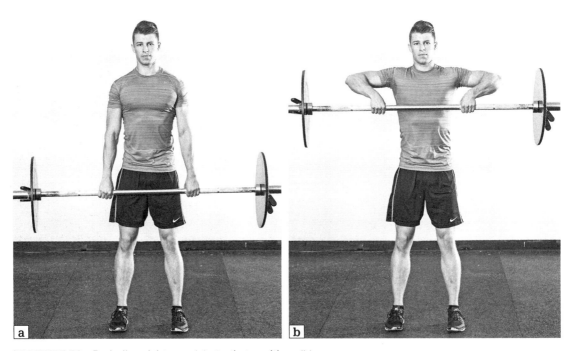

FIGURE 5.51 Barbell upright row: *(a)* starting position; *(b)* row.

Conclusion

Chapters 4 and 5 provide a comprehensive collection of exercises that allow the design of functional training programs for various sports. With the inclusion of traditional exercises, it is possible to integrate functional and traditional training to get the most out of training. Now we are ready for the programming portion of this book, and part III begins this process. In the next chapter, we discuss the theory and methods of periodization.

PART III

Programs

CHAPTER 6

Program Design

Periodization is a big word in the world of strength and conditioning. It is a theoretical training model that organizes training variables over a specific length of time. The reasons for organizing and manipulating training variables are to avoid overtraining and to peak an athlete at a specific point in time. Although many coaches and athletes know of periodization, there are still many who don't know how to create periodized strength programs. Periodization is even more confusing when it comes to functional training, which has not been universally defined and is hard to quantify. This chapter covers the concept of periodization and how to apply it to traditional training and functional training alike. Applying periodization to functional training can lead to unprecedented athleticism, and the surface has yet to be scratched in terms of the strength that periodized functional training can develop.

Training Variables

The two main training variables in periodization are volume and intensity. Volume can be expressed in total repetitions (sets × repetitions) or total tonnage (repetitions × weight lifted). We will use the most common expression: total repetitions. In the beginning stages of training, volume is high. This allows athletes to practice and to develop efficient movement. In addition, it gives the connective tissues time to remodel and become stronger. As the training progresses, volume drops to allow the second variable, intensity, to come into play.

Intensity refers to the load of an exercise and has an inverse relationship with volume. Although various factors can influence load, intensity usually involves the weight used, or the resistance the body moves against. At the beginning of training, when volume is high, intensity is low. The lighter loads allow for more repetitions and a greater volume of work during the initial stages of training. As the training progresses over weeks or months, the volume of work decreases while the intensity of training increases (see figure 6.1).

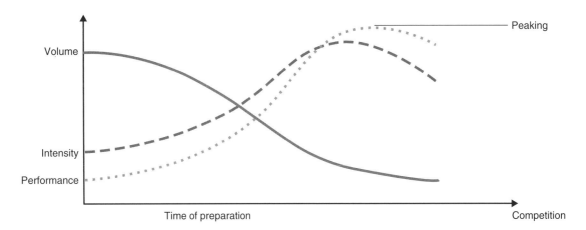

FIGURE 6.1 Periodization model.

Other important variables to consider are frequency and duration of training. However, these variables are also methods of expressing volume and manipulating intensity. For example, an athlete who needs a high volume may spread the work over more training sessions throughout the day, reducing the volume of work at each training session while increasing overall volume. This high frequency reduces the time for recovery, and thus the intensity must be significantly lower to avoid overtraining. Conversely, if higher training intensities are needed, the duration of the training session must be reduced to sustain the higher work and power output.

Periodization Cycles

Periodization manipulates training volume, intensity, and related variables over time and organizes them into four phases (or cycles): (1) the hypertrophy or conditioning phase, (2) the strength phase, (3) the power phase, and (4) the power-endurance phase. The four phases of periodization take the same approach to developing an athlete's physiology that a builder takes to building a house (see figure 6.2). First, a solid foundation must be laid (i.e., conditioning or hypertrophy phase). Second, the walls must be erected on the solid foundation (i.e., strength phase). Third, the roof is built on the strong and stable walls (i.e., power phase). Fourth, the doors and windows are finished to make the house fully functional (i.e., power-endurance phase). Let's talk about the specific intensities of each periodization phase and how they affect the exercises selected in each phase.

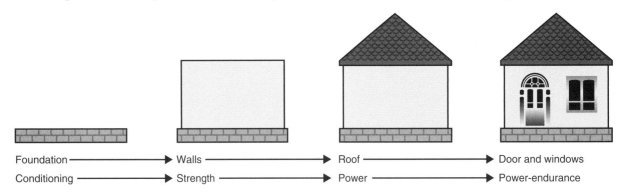

FIGURE 6.2 Building the house of periodization.

Assigning Loads and Intensities

Many athletes assign loads based on the amount of weight they can lift in a single repetition, known as the *1-repetition max*, or simply the *1RM*. All phases of periodization are assigned a percentage of this 1RM as the load to use during that specific phase. This can be one of the most confusing and cumbersome approaches to take when assigning loads, plus it makes it impossible to periodize functional training.

The problems with this approach are numerous. To start, 1RM can change daily or weekly due to a variety of reasons, from mood to amount of sleep to diet to increases in strength due to the rapid neural learning that takes place early in training. It is not practical to test for a 1RM on each exercise daily or weekly, so the numbers of a 1RM can be way off at any point during training. Assigning a percentage of an incorrect number will result in an incorrect load. For this reason I haven't used the percentage-of-1RM method since the 1990s.

The 1RM has been closely estimated using a multiple-repetition extrapolation. This method not only allows you to estimate the 1RM, but you can also estimate the percentage of the 1RM (table 6.1). Using the repetitions assigned to each percentage of the 1RM is the easiest way to train at the right intensity without worrying about the exact value of the 1RM. It eliminates all of the problems associated with the ever-changing 1RM and any corresponding percentage of it. Using the scale in table 6.1, you would simply choose a load that you could lift for 6 reps if you wanted to train in the 85 percent range of the predicted 1RM value.

TABLE 6.1 Percentage of 1RM Repetition Scale

Percentage of repetition maximum (%1RM)	Maximal repetitions
100%	1
95%	2
90%	4
85%	6
80%	8
75%	10
70%	12
65%	14
60%	16

Estimating repetitions not only avoids the 1RM measuring ordeal, it also allows you to assign intensity values to exercises for which a 1RM is impossible to measure, such as the single-leg squat. Using the repetition estimate and a little knowledge about functional training, we can periodize functional training using well-founded scientific principles. For example, if you wanted to work at 80 percent intensity on a push-up, you would simply manipulate the lever arm, the base, or the range of motion of the push to make it hard enough that you could only complete about 8 repetitions.

When working with weight, selecting the loads is easy; you simply move the pin to the correct weight or adjust the weight on a bar. However, when it comes to functional training, objectively manipulating loads is not so simple. You need to use more subjective measures. Let's take a look at how to approach exercise selection and use the concept of progression to program any phase of periodization using functional training.

Using the chest as an example, we can examine how traditional strength training views the choice of loading parameters and how that differs from loading and intensity in functional training modalities. If a strong athlete were going to select an exercise to provide high-intensity strength training for the chest during the strength phase, the bench press or chest machine would be likely choices. To select a strength intensity, the athlete would probably choose a load corresponding to 85 to 90 percent of 1RM, or 4 to 6 maximal repetitions. Using traditional training methods, loading a machine to a specific load is as easy as changing a pin or loading plates on a bar. However, what happens if this athlete wants to use functional training to provide the same training intensity to the chest? In the old days it was thought that functional training could not be periodized because the loads could not be quantified and manipulated, especially at higher intensities. Now we know better.

Using functional progression, any functional exercise can be manipulated to the desired training intensity. The strong athlete in our example can get excellent training for the chest using a progression of various functional chest exercises, such as the push-up. Even if this athlete could pump out 20 or more bodyweight push-ups, we could approximate the intensity of 4 to 6 repetitions (i.e., 85-90 percent 1RM) with a progression of the MB single-arm push-off (chapter 5). This approach can be used for any body part and functional progression. Using the tweaks discussed earlier in this book (e.g., base, lever arm, speed, range of motion), any functional exercise can be modified to the appropriate training intensity.

For the reasons stated in this section and many more, for the remainder of this text we will use the multiple-repetition method of assigning intensities and loads throughout each training phase. Remember that the percentages chosen to train during the phases of periodization, the measure of 1RM, and the information in table 6.1 are guidelines for making your training effective yet easy. The last thing I want to do is turn your training into a nightmare of calculations and measurements. Now, let's take a look at each phase of periodization.

Conditioning or Hypertrophy Phase

The conditioning (or hypertrophy) phase is the most common phase where athletes stay stuck for years. If you ask an athlete how many sets and reps she does of an exercise, the most common answer you will get is 3 to 5 sets of 10 reps. This is probably the most common range of sets and repetitions for developing hypertrophy, which is why conditioning and hypertrophy are grouped in the same phase and we use the terms synonymously when it comes to periodization.

The most distinguishing attribute of the conditioning phase is the volume of work completed in each workout or throughout the week. In this phase, the volume of work is the highest. The high volume characteristic of the conditioning phase provides a lot of repetitions. From a hypertrophy standpoint, the repetitive microtrauma of muscle fibers and subsequent remodeling require high volume and time for the hypertrophic response to occur. From a functional standpoint, the high number of repetitions typical in high-volume training is necessary for the biomotor learning needed to execute movements with precision.

Although various methods and strategies may be used to assign weekly volume of training during the conditioning phase, I have found that 12 to 20 sets of 8 to 15 repetitions per body system (e.g., legs, chest, back) are effective for developing a training base and hypertrophy if desired. For example, if an athlete wanted to develop a conditioning program for the legs and hips, the program would include a weekly volume of 12 to 20 sets for the legs, and each set would contain 8 to 15 repetitions, or a generic range of 10 to 20 repetitions. This program could be set up in a variety of ways (see table 6.2). As you can see in the table, the total weekly training volume for the legs is 12 to 15 sets. It does not matter how your

TABLE 6.2   Traditional and Functional Approaches to Weekly Conditioning for the Legs

TRADITIONAL APPROACH	
One day per week	**Three days per week**
Monday:	**Monday:**
Barbell squat	Barbell squat
4 or 5 × 15	4 or 5 × 15
Loaded alternating lunge (DB)	**Wednesday:**
4 or 5 × 10 per side	Loaded alternating lunge (DB)
Barbell deadlift	4 or 5 × 10 per side
4 or 5 × 15	**Friday:**
	Barbell deadlift
	4 or 5 × 15

FUNCTIONAL APPROACH	
One day per week	**Three days per week**
Monday:	**Monday:**
KB single-arm swing	KB single-arm swing
4 or 5 × 15	4 or 5 × 15
DB or KB lateral reaching lunge	**Wednesday:**
4 or 5 × 10 per side	DB or KB lateral reaching lunge
BP deadlift	4 or 5 × 10 per side
4 or 5 × 15	**Friday:**
	BP deadlift
	4 or 5 × 15

legs get the weekly training volume as long as they get it. However, taking a rest day between leg days is recommended.

As you can see, the conditioning phase is one of patience, learning, high repetitions, and lots of work. This high-volume training provides a solid foundation on which to build the second phase of periodization—strength.

Strength Phase

Strength may be the predominant theme in traditional strength training. A common training question is, "What's your bench?" However, functional strength has not traditionally approached strength from a high-intensity perspective. Instead its focus has been on repetitive functional movements so that the big strength developed in the traditional lifts could somehow be transferred to functional movement. In this section, I break that tradition and provide insight into how to design the strength phase using traditional methods as well as functional training.

In contrast to the conditioning phase, the predominant variable during the strength phase is intensity. High-intensity, low-volume training encapsulates the strength phase. This is accomplished primarily through the use of high training loads and low repetitions. Whereas the high volume of the conditioning and hypertrophy phase is taxing on the muscle fibers and metabolic systems, strength training is more taxing on the central nervous system. Because the volume is low, the muscle doesn't stay under loads for long, but the high level of neural impulses and recruitment of motor units make this an energy-intensive training period. Also, in contrast to the conditioning and hypertrophy phase, where full recovery between sets is not used, the high neural demands of the strength phase require greater recovery levels and thus longer rest periods. The strength phase is not about the grind; it's about taking your time, pushing big loads, and taking your central nervous system output to a higher level.

The effective weekly volume during a strength phase is 10 to 12 sets per week of 4 to 6 repetitions per body system (e.g., legs, chest, back). For example, an athlete who has gone through the hypertrophy phase and is interested in developing strength in the chest would plan a weekly volume of 10 to 12 sets for the chest, with each set containing only 4 to 6 repetitions, or a generic range of about 5 repetitions. This program could spread the volume of work throughout the week using one day, two days, or three days. Table 6.3 shows an example of a single-day program and a three-day program. As you can see, the total weekly training volume for the chest using a functional approach is 9 to 12 sets. As was the case with conditioning, it does not matter how the chest gets the weekly training volume as long as it gets it. Again, a rest day between chest strength days is highly recommended.

The strength phase is where functional training can shine and come out of its movement training and rehab stereotypes. Everyone is used to seeing func-

TABLE 6.3 Traditional and Functional Approaches to Weekly Functional Strength for the Chest

TRADITIONAL APPROACH

One day per week	Three days per week
Monday: Barbell flat bench press 3 or 4 × 4 to 6 reps Barbell incline bench press 3 or 4 × 4 to 6 reps Barbell overhead press 3 or 4 × 4 to 6 reps	**Monday:** Barbell flat bench press 3 or 4 × 4 to 6 reps **Wednesday:** Barbell incline bench press 3 or 4 × 4 to 6 reps **Friday:** Barbell overhead press 3 or 4 × 4 to 6 reps

FUNCTIONAL APPROACH
(GORILLA STRENGTH TRAINING)

One day per week	Three days per week
Monday: Weighted dip 3 or 4 × 4 to 6 reps BP staggered-stance CLA press 3 or 4 × 4 to 6 reps per side MB single-arm push-off 3 or 4 × 4 to 6 reps per side	**Monday:** Weighted dip 3 or 4 × 4 to 6 reps **Wednesday:** BP staggered-stance CLA press 3 or 4 × 4 to 6 reps per side **Friday:** MB single-arm push-off 3 or 4 × 4 to 6 reps per side

tional training at a moderate intensity or seeing more difficult moves performed for 5 to 10 repetitions. However, deliberately programming intense functional exercises for strength repetition ranges of 4 to 6 throughout an entire strength phase has not been common. In fact, I have never seen it in any literature or in any other training system. I have been experimenting with this application for approximately 10 years. I call the strength phase with functional training *gorilla strength training*. The reason for the name is obvious; my athletes get gorilla strong, or farmer strong, if you prefer. If you give this approach a chance, you will see your functional strength reach amazing levels, all without touching a piece of traditional equipment.

The strength phase is about quality high-intensity training. This is not the time to get in shape with incomplete recovery training. If you want to keep some level of conditioning, you can perform interval training after your strength training. For example, try three to five 30-second hits on a VersaClimber at about 200 to 250 feet (61 m) per minute with 1 to 2 minutes of rest in between. Strength training requires concentration, high neural input, and good recovery. Paying attention to the details of this phase will set the stage for the speed-dominated exercises of the upcoming power phase.

Power Phase

Power training can be exciting and offer quick returns for the time invested. But before we talk about programming for power, let's clear up the misconceptions surrounding power training. Understanding what power training is and what it is not will better help you understand the programming aspect of this training mode.

Misconceptions About Power Training

There are many ways to train for power, from Olympic weightlifting to medicine ball throws to plyometrics. An enormous amount of confusion surrounds power training, so it would be beneficial to draw some distinctions between various methods of developing power. Power is defined by these equations:

$$\text{Power} = \text{force} \times \text{speed}$$
$$\text{Power} = \text{work} / \text{time}$$

The first equation shows why speed is an important factor of power. The loads must be light enough for the athlete to be able to move with speed. One of the main misconceptions is about the proper loading for functional power. If you look at the loads of functional sport movements, you will notice that they are light. Gloves, balls, bats, rackets, and clubs weigh ounces, not tens or hundreds of pounds. Therefore, an athlete's functional sport power develops using high speed at low loads. It's a mistake to think that high-power readings on specialized equipment are the final end game in power development. What some of this equipment does is make an athlete better at moving heavier weights than would be found in the athlete's sport. Additionally, these heavier loads are moved at speeds that are slower than those found in the sport. Therefore, power training needs to progress from heavier loads in the strength phase to lighter loads in the power phase. The lighter loads and faster speeds of the power phase allow the athlete to concentrate on sport speed.

Another misconception is that power training is plyometric training. All plyometric training is power training, but not all power training is plyometric training. The difference is that some power training, such as a vertical jump from a squat, does not use the myotatic reflex typical of plyometric training. To invoke the myotatic reflex, there needs to be a fast stretching of the tendons of the leg and hip muscles, such as during a depth jump, when the athlete jumps off one box, rebounds off the ground, and jumps onto another box. Even the counter-movement before a vertical jump does not provide enough speed to invoke the myotatic reflex that the depth jump does. The same goes for a medicine ball chest throw and repetitive explosive push-up. The chest throw makes for effective power training, but the stretch reflex is not fast enough to be plyometric, unlike the repetitive explosive push-up. Effective power training does not have to be plyometric; both plyometric and nonplyometric power exercises are successful at developing power. I would even venture to say that nonplyometric power exercise yields excellent results without the wear and tear associated with heavy plyometric training. When dealing with younger and heavier athletes, I mostly use nonplyometric power exercises for power development.

Programming of Power

The power phase is the most exciting phase of training. It's exciting because this is where power improvements look as dramatic as they feel. This is when athletes start to see improvements in running speed, bat and club speed, ball speed, jump height, and changes in direction. That's why many athletes start doing power training without a base. However, similar to building a house without the proper foundation, power training without the proper foundation will lead to substandard results and possible injury.

Similar to the strength phase, the volume of work is low during the power phase. Training speed reaches an all-time high during the power phase. Like strength training, power training is demanding on the neural system, requires full recovery, and focuses on quality movement and all-out efforts. Unlike hypertrophy and strength training, the contractions used in power training are of short duration, which means the training is not taxing on the muscle fibers or metabolic system. However, the speed of the contraction during power training is fast, putting enormous demands on the central nervous system. Athletes feel relaxed after power training, not tired. This sensation of being relaxed is the exhaustion of the central nervous system kicking in.

As mentioned, the volume of work in the power phase is similar to the volume in the strength phase. Eight to 12 sets per week of approximately 5 repetitions of a traditional exercise coupled with 5 repetitions of an explosive equivalent per body system (e.g., legs, chest, back) is an effective range. As with the other phases, the volume can be spread out over the week, or all of the power training for a body system can be done on a single day. This may not seem like a lot of work, but when you exert maximal effort for every repetition in a workout, 40 reps seem like an eternity and leave you ready for a nap. As usual, a rest day between power days for a specific body part is highly recommended.

There are many approaches to programming workouts during the power phase. You can perform power exercises at the beginning of a strength workout, have a dedicated power day in which the entire workout consists of power exercises, or combine strength and power exercises to create power complexes. All three methods are worth further discussion.

In the first scenario, we can add sets of medicine ball throws and explosive push-ups before a chest strength workout. The workout can be performed two times per week and might look like this:

Monday and Wednesday

Beginners start with 3 sets and slowly proceed to 4 or 5 sets.

MB staggered-stance CLA straight chest throw 4 or 5 × 5

Explosive push-up 4 or 5 × 5

Any strength exercise for the chest 4 to 6 × 4 to 6

For the second option, a dedicated power day can address the entire body or a specific body system. A total-body workout can include 4 or 5 sets of a lower-body exercise, a push exercise, a pull exercise, and a rotational exercise, and it can be performed two days per week. The following program illustrates this:

Monday and Wednesday

Beginners start with 3 sets and slowly proceed to 4 or 5 sets.

Vertical jump 4 or 5 × 5

MB crossover push-up 4 or 5 × 5

MB overhead slam 4 or 5 × 5

MB rotational throw: perpendicular 4 or 5 × 5

The third option for programming a power workout is to use one of the most exciting methods we have found—the complex training method. Dr. Donald Chu brought this method to the mainstream of strength and conditioning with the publication of *Explosive Power and Strength* in 1996. In this text, Dr. Chu extensively covers the history, science, and practice of combining strength training and power training. I have simplified this method to complexes that anyone can do anywhere with little equipment.

Here is the premise:

- Perform 5 hard repetitions of a strength exercise.
- Rest 1 minute.
- Perform 5 repetitions of an explosive equivalent exercise that is biomechanically similar to the strength exercise (i.e., uses the same muscle systems and movement).

The idea is to load the muscle enough to excite the neural components but not metabolically fatigue them. Then, take a brief rest that allows the muscle to recover but takes advantage of the central nervous system excitation. Finally, perform the explosive equivalent. This approach results in more power expression in the explosive equivalent exercise as a result of the neural excitation caused by the previous strength exercise. A power complex using conventional methods of strength training can look like this:

- Perform 5 repetitions of a bench press.
- Rest 1 minute.
- Perform 5 repetitions of an explosive push-up.

A power complex using purely functional training can look like this:

- Perform 5 repetitions of a right-handed BP staggered-stance CLA press.
- Rest 1 minute.
- Perform 5 repetitions of a right-handed MB staggered-stance CLA straight chest throw.

An additional advantage of the complex method of power development is that a strength component is trained when the heavy strength exercise is performed. This maintains strength levels during the power phase and also allows for reducing the strength phase if time is short. During emergencies and with athletes who have a good training base, the strength phase can be skipped and the athlete can do the power phase because of the strength training inherent in the complex method.

Tables 6.4 and 6.5 illustrate sample power complexes over a week.

Power-Endurance Phase

The power-endurance phase of training is when the athlete creates the power endurance necessary to outlast the competition. Challenging metabolic circuits and prefatigue strategies take the athlete's neural and metabolic systems to an

TABLE 6.4 Weekly Power Complex:
Traditional and Functional Training Combined

TOTAL BODY (MONDAY AND WEDNESDAY)

Exercise	Sets and reps
Barbell squat and vertical jump	3 × 5 + 5
Barbell flat bench press and explosive push-up	3 × 5 + 5
Seated cable row and MB overhead slam throw	3 × 5 + 5

SPLIT HYBRID (MONDAY, WEDNESDAY, FRIDAY)

Exercise	Sets and reps	Exercise	Sets and reps	Exercise	Sets and reps
Barbell squat Vertical jump	3 × 5 + 5	Barbell flat bench press Explosive push-up	3 × 5 + 5	Seated cable row MB overhead side-to-side slam	3 × 5 + 5
Loaded alternating lunge (DB) Alternating split jump	3 × 5 + 5	Barbell incline bench press MB staggered-stance CLA incline chest throw	3 × 5 + 5	Pull-down MB overhead slam	3 × 5 + 5
Barbell deadlift Burpee	3 × 5 + 5	Weighted dip MB staggered-stance CLA decline chest throw	3 × 5 + 5	Barbell upright row MB reverse scoop throw	3 × 5 + 5

5 + 5 indicates five repetitions of the first exercise, 60 seconds of rest, and five repetitions of the second exercise.

TABLE 6.5 Weekly Power Complex: Functional Training Only

TOTAL BODY
(MONDAY AND WEDNESDAY)

Exercise	Sets and reps
Single-leg squat Single-leg push-off	3 × 5 + 5
MB single-arm push-off MB staggered-stance CLA straight chest throw	3 × 5 + 5
Recline pull MB overhead slam	3 × 5 + 5

SPLIT HYBRID (MONDAY, WEDNESDAY, FRIDAY)

Exercise	Sets and reps	Exercise	Sets and reps	Exercise	Sets and reps
Single-leg squat Single-leg push-off	3 × 5 + 5*	BP staggered-stance CLA incline chest press MB staggered-stance CLA incline chest throw	3 × 5 + 5	Recline pull MB overhead slam	3 × 5 + 5
Alternating split jump (DB) Alternating split jump (body weight)	3 × 5 + 5	MB single-arm push-off MB staggered-stance CLA straight chest throw	3 × 5 + 5	BP staggered-stance CLA row MB overhead side-to-side slam	3 × 5 + 5
BP deadlift Vertical jump	3 × 5 + 5	BP staggered-stance CLA decline chest press MB staggered-stance CLA decline chest throw	3 × 5 + 5	BP staggered-stance CLA low-to-high row MB reverse scoop throw	3 × 5 + 5

5 + 5 indicates five repetitions of the first exercise, 60 seconds of rest, and five repetitions of the second exercise.

all-time high. Although this is the most energy-intensive phase, proper periodization prepares the athlete for its demands.

Power endurance can be programmed in many ways, but I have found two strategies to be the most effective. One strategy involves complex training, similar to that of the power phase. The other strategy uses metabolic circuits. I have even developed programs that combine both strategies in an efficient and entertaining way. Let's take a look at how you can use each strategy to develop power endurance.

The first strategy for programming power endurance is identical in format to the complex training discussed in the power section. However, to work on endurance, I eliminate the 1-minute rest between the strength exercise and the subsequent explosive equivalent. This power training with incomplete recovery allows the strength exercise to serve not only as a neural excitation stimulus but also as a prefatigue modality. The subsequent power exercise provides the power endurance implied by the name of this training phase. Taking the previous complex used for power training, the power-endurance complex is reduced to the following protocols.

Using Traditional Strength and Power Training

- Perform 5 hard repetitions of a strength exercise, such as the barbell squat.
- Skip the rest period.
- Perform 5 to 10 repetitions of an explosive equivalent of the strength exercise, such as the vertical jump.

Using Functional Training Exclusively

- Perform 5 repetitions of a functional strength exercise, such as the MB single-arm push-off.
- Skip the rest period.
- Perform 5 to 10 repetitions of an explosive equivalent of the functional strength exercise, such as the MB staggered-stance CLA straight chest throw.

When programming the power complexes in the power-endurance phase, use volume identical to that used in the power phase. Employ this training for 8 to 12 sets per week of the 5+5 repetitions scheme for each body part (e.g., legs, chest, back). It is fine to experiment with the number of repetitions of the explosive equivalents, depending on the sport you're preparing for. I have used up to 10 repetitions of the explosive equivalent for endurance sports such as cross country running. The volume can be spread out over the week, or all of the power training for a body system can be done on a single day. A rest day between training days of a specific body part is recommended.

The next strategy for developing power endurance is metabolic circuits (see chapter 7). These circuits consist of three to eight exercises that are each performed for 10 to 30 repetitions or for time (e.g., 15-60 seconds). A metabolic circuit can concentrate on one body part (e.g., JC Leg Crank) or can mimic a specific sport scenario (e.g., 5-minute MMA circuits).

JC Leg Crank

Bodyweight double-leg squat × 24

Bodyweight alternating lunge × 24 (12/leg)

Alternating split jump × 24 (12/leg)

Squat jump × 12

Total circuit time: 1:20 to 1:30

MMA Circuit

Mat sprawl × 20

Gable hang 30 sec.

DB punch × 30

Sling curl × 30

MB V-up exchange × 20

Get-up × 10

Short cable double-hand pull × 30

Low kick × 10 per leg

Low punch × 30

Total circuit time: 5:00 to 6:00

These metabolic circuits provide incredible power endurance and can be used in a variety of ways. You can use the metabolic protocols as a flush set at the end of a bodybuilding or strength workout to provide extra blood to the area worked or to develop a base level of endurance in preparation for the power-endurance phase. For example, you can perform 1 to 3 sets of JC Leg Crank at the end of a leg workout, 1 or 2 sets of JC Meta Chest at the end of a chest workout, and 1 or 2 sets of JC Meta Back (see chapter 7) at the end of a total-body workout.

Another strategy to implement metabolic protocols is to use them as a prefatigue method for sport-specific training. For example, 1 to 4 sets of the JC Leg Crank can prefatigue a marathon runner before doing a 5- to 10-mile (8-16 km) run. This allows the marathon runner to experience what it feels like to run long distances without ever having to run the long distance. Additionally, the metabolic protocols can provide well-needed strength for sports that traditionally have not used strength programs, all without setting foot in a gym. This prefatigue approach adds strength training to endurance sports, cuts down training volume, and reduces overtraining injuries.

Finally, metabolic protocols that mimic sport-play metabolics, such as fighting circuits, can provide better conditioning than actually playing the sport, without the risk of injury associated with intense practice and overuse. This application is particularly useful for sports that have high injury rates, such as combat sports. For example, fighting circuits such as the MMA circuit can replace live sparring as a conditioning strategy or at least prefatigue a few rounds so that a fighter can reduce the rounds sparred.

Using metabolic protocols to provide power endurance, prefatigue training, or substitute training can reduce traditional training volume by as much as 50 percent. It can also reduce overtraining injuries while producing personal best performances in athletes.

Putting It All Together

The ideal length of each periodization phase has been much debated. Some books provide ranges from 3 weeks to 8 weeks. I prefer to keep each phase to about 4 weeks. This provides a block of training that covers all four phases and brings an athlete to a peak over 16 weeks. In a 52-week year, an athlete can peak three times, with some time off between each peak.

Sometimes competition schedules do not fall into neat 16-week time slots. In these cases, there are three main strategies for manipulating the periodization timeline. The first strategy is to not train what is not needed. This means if an athlete is already big enough, don't bother with the hypertrophy phase. Likewise, if an athlete plays a power sport, such as golf, don't spend time in the power-endurance phase. This strategy can take weeks or months off the total program time. For example, let's consider a baseball player who is already big and does not need power endurance. His program might have 4 weeks in the strength phase and 4 weeks in the power phase, assuming he already has a good conditioning base. This strategy would save 8 weeks from the standard 16-week timeline.

The second strategy is to shorten the cycles that are needed the least. This prioritizes the training and allows the athlete to spend more time on the attributes needed. For example, let's say we need to train a wrestler in 7 weeks. First, a wrestler does not need more muscle mass, and power endurance is the attribute to concentrate on. A sound approach would be to spend 1 week on conditioning to create a base, 1 week on strength, 1 week on power, and 4 weeks on power endurance to make sure he is in shape to wrestle. It may seem that 1-week cycles will not do much, but when faced with difficult circumstances and short time periods, you must work with what you have, however imperfect it may be.

The third strategy is to blend or combine phases. This approach acknowledges that the conditioning and strength phases are practically the same and only change the volume of the training (i.e., sets and reps). Likewise, the complexes used in the power and power-endurance phases only differ in the rest periods between the strength and power exercises within each complex (table 6.6).

Using the 7-week wrestling program as an example, we can combine the conditioning and strength phase to 2 weeks and the power and power endurance to 5 weeks.

TABLE 6.6 Combining Phases

Phase	Conditioning and strength		Power and power endurance				
Week	1	2	3	4	5	6	7
Reps of strength and power training exercises	8	6	5 + 5	5 + 5	5 + 5	5 +5	5 + 5
Rest between strength training and power exercise in complex	N/A	N/A	60 sec.	30 sec.	15 sec.	0 sec.	0 sec.

5 + 5 indicates five repetitions of the first exercise, 60 seconds of rest, and five repetitions of the second exercise.

Conclusion

We have covered just some of the many strategies for periodizing training and designing effective programs. The old adage, "Program design is as much an art as it is a science," is certainly true. Don't be afraid to experiment with various formats and strategies. However, always stay on the conservative side of new implementations. Also, consider consulting a strength and conditioning specialist certified by the National Strength and Conditioning Association (NSCA CSCS) or a trainer or performance coach certified by IHP University (IHPU) for proper execution of movements and sound programming. Safety and effectiveness should be the top priorities when programming for sport-specific function.

CHAPTER 7

Pure Functional Training

This chapter provides everything an athlete needs to train for any sport. The programs presented here can serve multiple purposes; they can create a modest training base, train specific athletic attributes, and supplement other programs. They can also be used when not a lot of time is available for training (e.g., in-season, travel). Regardless of how you use these programs, the key characteristics of each are simplicity, ease of use, and effectiveness. Even the express programs can yield huge benefits with just minutes of training a few times per week.

The training programs in this chapter and in chapter 9 represent both a general and specific approach to functional training for sport. General conditioning and the most popular sport skills and sport categories are covered for the widest possible application. Because each sport may have various positions that require completely different qualities, some of the express protocols deal with specific sport qualities. For example, you can add the speed-demon program to any sport program to improve running speed. These express programs provide more specificity and variety to the already robust programming options presented in this book.

The functional strength exercises in the following programs develop strength in general movement patterns associated with various sport drills. They build the strength to improve your sport-specific training using ladder drills, cone drills, resisted sport skills, and other sport-specific movements. Combining functional training with a sport-specific program results in the ultimate transfer from exercise to sport skill.

Integrating Functional Training Into Your Training Plan

Each sport-specific program in chapter 9 includes three types of workouts: a conditioning day, a strength day, and a power or power-endurance day. A beginning athlete should perform the conditioning day two or three times per week for two to four weeks and then move on to the strength program. An athlete with at least a month of base training can start with the strength workout and perform it two or three times per week for two to four weeks before proceeding to the power program. An experienced and conditioned athlete with plenty of strength who is looking for power development can start with the power workout two or three times per week for two to four weeks and then proceed to the power-endurance program if needed. An experienced and conditioned athlete who is looking for power endurance can perform the power-endurance workouts two or three times per week for two to four weeks. Finally, some advanced athletes prefer to use an undulating method of training in which day 1 is a conditioning day, day 2 is a strength day, and day 3 is a power or power-endurance day. This undulating format can be performed for a longer period (2-3 months), and a reduced version of this program can be used for in-season training.

To tailor the intensity of the exercises in the following programs, use the tweaks previously discussed in this book. This means manipulating the range of motion, lever arm, speed, base, and external load to make the assigned number of repetitions and sets challenging. For example, if you are assigned a dumbbell reaching lunge for 4 to 6 repetitions during a strength phase, use enough load to make the 4 to 6 repetitions challenging. Likewise, if push-ups are assigned for 4 to 6 repetitions during a strength phase, slow the movement to a speed at which 4 to 6 repetitions become challenging.

You can also vary the load and the equipment used to provide that load. This means if a bodyweight lunge is too easy, you can load it with dumbbells, kettlebells, a medicine ball, or any other external free weight. Likewise, if you are assigned a dumbbell reaching lunge, you can load it with a medicine ball instead of dumbbells. The load is the load, and the body does not know what you are carrying in your hands. The intensity of the movement is what it is important. Make sure it's an intensity that allows you to complete the program as outlined.

A day of rest between workouts is recommended. However, don't worry if you have to work out two days in a row on occasion. As long as you don't make it a habit, your body will recover during subsequent normal weeks of training. That's one of the great things about functional training—it spreads the work over many muscle systems so it does not damage a targeted muscle the way bodybuilding does. This is how gymnasts, baseball players, wrestlers, and many other athletes can do the same thing every day without days off. Now, let's take a look at the functional training programs that will change the way you perform forever.

Grab-and-Go Protocols

The grab-and-go protocols are preprogrammed protocols that can be used as basic workouts to get a beginner started in foundational training (i.e., JV Program) or to kick-start the conditioning phase of an intermediate and even advanced training program (i.e., Varsity Program). Regardless of the grab-and-go program you chose, it will give you an idea of how to start programming functional training. Feel free to experiment with any combination of exercises in this book using the template you see in these simple programs.

This general conditioning program (table 7.1) involves the eight bodyweight progressions and is perfect for the novice athlete who is starting an exercise program for the first time. It's also ideal for a young athlete (8-13 years old) who has never trained and is curious about improving athletic ability via strength and conditioning.

THE EXERCISES

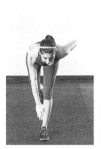

Single-leg CLA anterior reach.

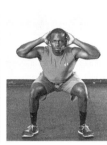

Single-leg squat.

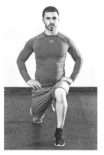

Bodyweight double-leg squat.

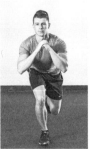

Bodyweight alternating lunge.

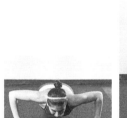

Bodyweight push-up.

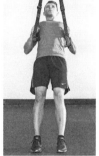

Recline pull (row).

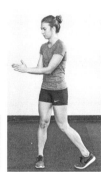

Rotation with pivot.

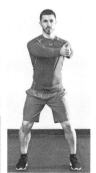

Rotation without pivot.

THE HOW

TABLE 7.1 JV Program

Perform this bodyweight program two or three times per week.

Exercise	Week 1	Week 2	Week 3	Week 4	Page
Single-leg CLA anterior reach	2 × 5 per side	2 × 10 per side	3 × 15 per side	4 × 20 per side	39
Single-leg squat	2 × 5 per side	2 × 7 per side	3 × 10 per side	4 × 10 per side	40
Bodyweight double-leg squat	2 × 10 per side	2 × 15 per side	3 × 15 per side	4 × 15 per side	42
Bodyweight alternating lunge	2 × 5 per side	2 × 10 per side	3 × 10 per side	4 × 10 per side	43
Bodyweight push-up	2 × 5	2 × 10	3 × 10	4 × 10	44
Recline pull (row)	2 × 5	2 × 10	3 × 10	4 × 10	46
Rotation with pivot	2 × 10 per side	2 × 15 per side	3 × 15 per side	4 × 20 per side	47
Rotation without pivot	2 × 10 per side	2 × 15 per side	3 × 15 per side	4 × 20 per side	48

The Varsity Program uses a variety of equipment to create an intermediate conditioning program (table 7.2) with more complex exercises than the JV Program. It's useful for a more experienced athlete who is returning from an injury or from off-season and is trying to get in shape for pre-season training (i.e., conditioning phase). A stronger athlete who has competed in sport but has never done formal strength training will also find this program useful. You can even get aggressive with this program and use heavy loads to keep the repetition range low (i.e., 4-6 reps), giving it more of a strength component during the strength phase for a novice or intermediate athlete.

THE EXERCISES

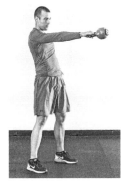

KB single-arm swing.

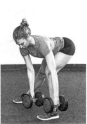

DB or KB lateral reaching lunge.

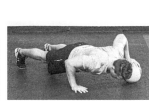

MB crossover push-up.

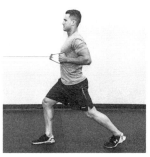

BP staggered-stance CLA row.

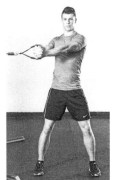

BP short rotation (10 to 2 o'clock).

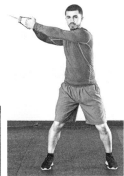

BP high-to-low chop.

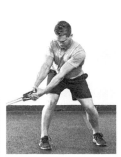

BP low-to-high chop.

THE HOW

TABLE 7.2 Varsity Program

Exercise	Week 1	Week 2	Week 3	Week 4	Page
KB single-arm swing	2 × 5 per side	2 × 10 per side	3 × 10 per side	4 × 10 per side	91
DB or KB lateral reaching lunge	2 × 5 per side	2 × 7 per side	3 × 10 per side	4 × 10 per side	95
MB crossover push-up	2 × 5 per side	2 × 7 per side	3 × 10 per side	4 × 10 per side	115
BP staggered-stance CLA row	2 × 10 per side	2 × 15 per side	3 × 15 per side	4 × 15 per side	81
BP short rotation (10 to 2 o'clock)	2 × 10 per side	2 × 10 per side	3 × 10 per side	4 × 10 per side	87
BP high-to-low chop	2 × 10 per side	2 × 10 per side	3 × 10 per side	4 × 10 per side	85
BP low-to-high chop	2 × 10 per side	2 × 10 per side	3 × 10 per side	4 × 10 per side	86

Express Protocols

The following protocols use specific training to improve a specific aspect of performance or a body part. They can be added to the sport-specific programs or serve as short workouts to stay in shape during short vacations or when full-time training is not possible. You can perform the exercises in a circuit or complete indicated sets of each exercise before going to the next. Performing these programs two or three times per week will provide noticeable results in as little as two weeks!

This program (table 7.3) is similar to the general Steel Core program presented later in the chapter but is tailored to improving backswing follow-through and the impact zone of the golfer. Combining this program with the Steel Core is an excellent way to improve your golf game.

THE EXERCISES

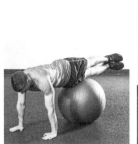

SB log roll.

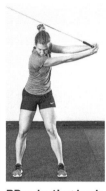

BP pulsating backswing.

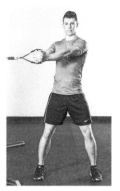

BP short rotation (10 to 2 o'clock).

THE HOW

TABLE 7.3 Golf Power-Drive Protocol

Exercise	Sets and reps	Page
SB log roll	3 × 10 to 15 per side	131
BP pulsating backswing	3 × 10 to 15 per side	88
BP short rotation (10 to 2 o'clock)	3 × 10 to 15 per side	87

This program (table 7.4) improves speed without running. You can perform this three-exercise complex during each commercial break of a TV show. That's why it's often referred to as the *TV Speed Program*.

THE EXERCISES

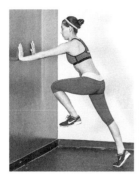
45-degree calf pump.

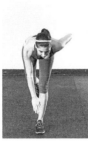
Single-leg CLA anterior reach.

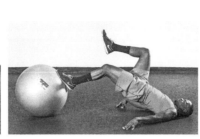
SB hip lift (single leg).

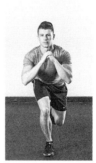
Single-leg squat.

THE HOW

TABLE 7.4 Running Speed-Demon Protocol

Exercise	Sets and reps	Page
45-degree calf pump (progress from double legs to single leg)	30 to 60 sec. (per side when on single leg)	63
Single-leg CLA anterior reach	3 × 10 to 15 per side	39
SB hip lift (single leg)	3 × 10 to 15 per side	128
Single-leg squat (quarter range of motion)	3 × 10 to 15 per side	142

This program (table 7.5) improves your punching power. It involves the unilateral pushing component found in punching, stiff-arming, and other pushing-related sport skills. Not only does it emphasize the pushing action, it also develops the rotational stiffness these skills require for maximum power generation.

THE EXERCISES

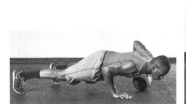
MB single-arm push-off.

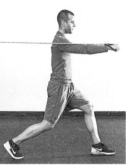
BP staggered-stance CLA press.

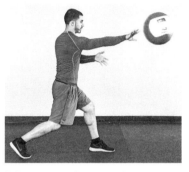
MB staggered-stance CLA straight chest throw.

THE HOW

TABLE 7.5 KO Protocol

Exercise	Sets and reps	Page
MB single-arm push-off	3 × 10 per side	114
BP staggered-stance CLA press	3 × 10 to 15 per side	72
MB staggered-stance CLA straight chest throw	3 × 5 to 10 per side	118

This program (table 7.6) improves the ability to cut on a dime, and it's excellent for skaters. It targets the ability of the glutes to extend while externally rotating. This a great protocol to perform at home, to use as a warm-up or cool-down for a workout, or to add to your current strength and conditioning program.

THE EXERCISES

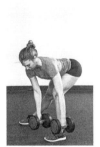

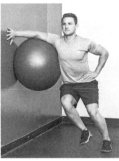

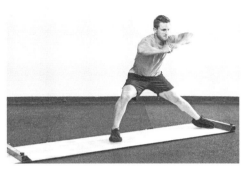

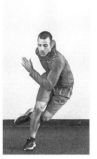

DB or KB lateral reaching lunge. **SB single-leg lateral wall slide.** Lateral slide. Skater.

THE HOW

TABLE 7.6   Cut Protocol

Exercise	Sets and reps	Page
DB or KB lateral reaching lunge	2 or 3 × 10 to 15 per side	95
SB single-leg lateral wall slide	2 or 3 × 10 to 15 per side	124
Lateral slide	2 or 3 × 5 to 10 per side	140
Skater	2 or 3 × 5 to 10 per side	67

This program (table 7.7) improves overhead activities, such as throwing a ball or serving overhead in tennis. You can perform this program anywhere there is enough room to slam a medicine ball. You can also use it as a warm-up or cool-down to a workout or add it to your current strength and conditioning program.

THE EXERCISES

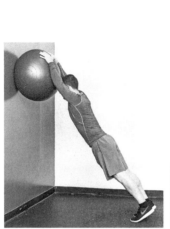

SB rollout.

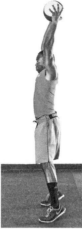

MB overhead slam.

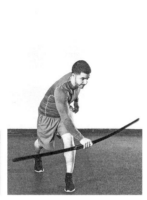

Vibration blade throw.

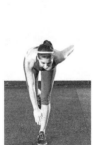

Single-leg CLA anterior reach.

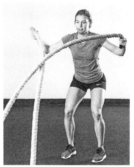

Rope circles (clockwise and counterclockwise).

THE HOW

TABLE 7.7 Flamethrower

Exercise	Sets and reps	Page
SB rollout	2 × 10 to 15	127
MB overhead slam	2 × 5 to 10	120
Vibration blade throw	2 × 10 to 15 sec. per side	133
Single-leg CLA anterior reach	2 × 10 to 15 per side	39
Rope circles (clockwise and counterclockwise)	2 × 10 to 15 sec. each direction	139

This program (table 7.8) improves batting power and is guaranteed to improve your batting average. You can perform it anywhere there is enough room to slam a medicine ball. You can also use it as a warm-up or cool-down to a workout or add it to your current strength and conditioning program.

THE EXERCISES

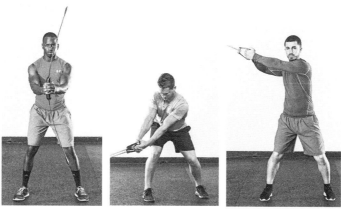

Vibration blade 12 o'clock oscillation.   **BP low-to-high chop.**   **BP high-to-low chop.**

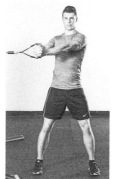 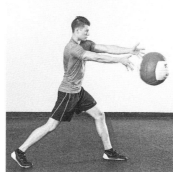

BP short rotation (10 to 2 o'clock).   **MB rotational throw: perpendicular.**

THE HOW

TABLE 7.8   Home-Run Protocol

Exercise	Sets and reps	Page
Vibration blade 12 o'clock oscillation	2 × 10 to 15 sec.	134
BP low-to-high chop	3 × 10 to 15 per side	86
BP high-to-low chop	3 × 10 to 15 per side	85
BP short rotation (10 to 2 o'clock)	3 × 10 to 15 per side	87
MB rotational throw: perpendicular	3 × 5 to 10 per side	121

General Fitness Protocols

You can use these short programs to strengthen a general area of the body or to develop general fitness or conditioning. They also make a great addition to any workout as a warm-up or cool-down. For example, the Core Activator (also known as the Short Chopper) has become a standard core warm-up, and the Triple Threat has become known as the Hamstrings of Steel program because it eliminates practically all hamstring problems.

Total-Body Training: Chopper

The Chopper program (table 7.9) is one of the most popular and diverse protocols at IHP. It epitomizes fingernail-to-toenail training. It is the most used warm-up among my athletes, and when heavy (25-45 lb [11-20 kg]) medicine balls or weight plates are used, it becomes a strength and conditioning protocol. Although the medicine ball version is outlined here, you can perform this protocol with any heavy implement, such as weight plates, sandbags, or a single dumbbell or kettlebell. For a great warm-up, use 3 to 6 pounds (1-3 kg). Large athletes can use 25 to 45 pounds (11-20 kg) to train total-body strength. You can perform this protocol as a circuit for warm-ups and conditioning work. For strength work, perform each exercise for the prescribed repetitions, and rest adequately between each set.

THE EXERCISES

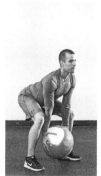 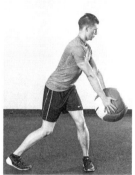 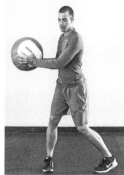

MB wood chop.   MB diagonal chop.   MB rotation with pivot.

THE HOW

TABLE 7.9 Chopper

Exercise	Sets and reps	Page
MB wood chop	3 × 10	110
MB diagonal chop	3 × 10 per side	111
MB rotation with pivot	3 × 10 per side	116

This program (table 7.10) is a variation of the Chopper minus the large ranges of motion at the lower body and hips. The Core Activator improves core stiffness without flexing the lower body, making it a perfect way to strengthen the core when a lower-body injury does not permit any squatting or lunging, or if you simply want to rest the lower body. I also use this protocol with light loads when starting to rehabilitate the lower back after an injury or surgery; it is a prehabilitator as well as a rehabilitator of the spine. You can use this protocol to warm up for a lower-body strength training workout or as a beginning conditioning protocol.

THE EXERCISES

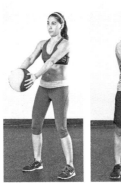 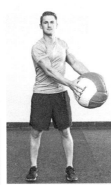 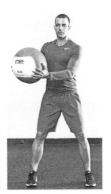

MB short wood chop.   MB short diagonal chop.   MB rotation without pivot.

THE HOW

TABLE 7.10   Core Activator

Exercise	Sets and reps	Page
MB short wood chop	3 × 10 per side	110
MB short diagonal chop	3 × 10 per side	112
MB rotation without pivot	3 × 10 per side	48

Core Stiffness: Steel Core

This program (table 7.11) is a version of the Chopper program with more direct and heavier loading through bands and pulleys. It creates core stiffness from the standing position while driving high-intensity loads to the diagonal and lateral musculature of the core. Athletes who use a stick for their sport can perform this protocol with a bar attached to a band or cable. This protocol can also be used to warm up or as an adjunct to the training of combat, court, and racket athletes. When training for strength, don't be afraid to go heavy. Use enough weight so the outside foot almost starts to come off the ground.

THE EXERCISES

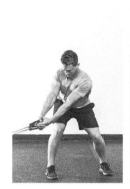
BP low-to-high chop.

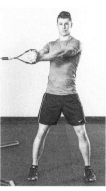
BP short rotation (10 to 2 o'clock).

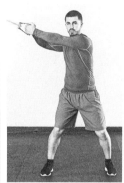
BP high-to-low chop.

THE HOW

TABLE 7.11 Steel Core

Exercise	Sets and reps	Page
BP low-to-high chop	3 × 10 per side	86
BP short rotation (10 to 2 o'clock)	3 × 10 per side	87
BP high-to-low chop	3 × 10 per side	85

This program (table 7.12) is excellent for total-body stability and strength. It also makes a great warm-up, cool-down, recovery, and functional training maintenance program during heavy-work hypertrophy or strength cycles. The sequence of the five exercises allows you to flow from one to the other—perfect for a continuous circuit. I love this protocol as a cool-down for big athletes who are concentrating on hypertrophy for a few weeks; 3 or 4 sets at the end of a workout keeps the core engaged.

THE EXERCISES

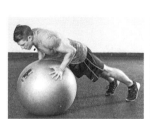 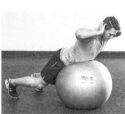 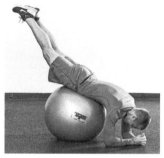

SB hands-on-ball push-up.   SB hyperextension.   SB reverse hyperextension.

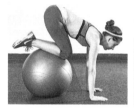 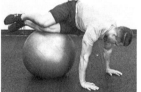

SB knee tuck (double leg to single leg).   SB skier.

THE HOW

TABLE 7.12   Fabulous Five

Perform the exercises in the sequence shown.

Exercise	Sets and reps	Page
SB hands-on-ball push-up	3 × 10	125
SB hyperextension	3 × 10	130
SB reverse hyperextension	3 × 10	131
SB knee tuck (double leg to single leg)	3 × 10 (per side when on single leg)	126
SB skier	3 × 10 per side	132

Hamstring Program: Triple Threat

Although this program (table 7.13) is not performed while standing, it improves hamstring strength and function. The Triple Threat is so effective as a hamstring rehabilitation and high-performance program that I call it the *Hamstrings of Steel* program. This protocol has saved the careers of many of my athletes who suffered from chronic hamstring injuries. You can use this protocol on off-days or as a cool-down after any workout.

Begin with the double-leg version of each exercise for weeks 1 through 10. Switch to the single-leg version of each exercise for weeks 11 through 20. Perform the protocol as a sequence with rest and without putting your hips on the ground—perform the bridges for the number of repetitions prescribed, keep your hips elevated and perform the leg curls for the number of repetitions prescribed, and finally keep your hips elevated and perform the hip lifts for the number of repetitions prescribed.

When performing the single-leg version of each exercise, use the free leg to maneuver or walk the stability ball into the next position without putting your hips on the ground.

THE EXERCISES

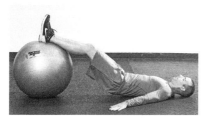
SB bridge.

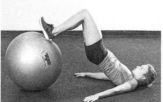
SB leg curl.

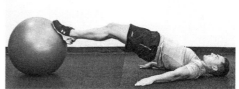
SB hip lift.

THE HOW

Double-leg version: In week 1, perform 5 reps of each exercise without resting or putting your hips on the ground. Add 1 rep of each exercise per week for 10 weeks. By week 10, you should be able to perform 15 reps of each exercise (45 total) without rest.

Single-leg version: In week 11, perform 5 reps of each exercise per leg without resting or putting your hips on the ground. Add 1 rep of each exercise per week for 10 weeks. By week 20, you should be able to perform 15 reps of each exercise (45 total) without rest.

TABLE 7.13 Triple Threat

Exercise	Weeks 1 through 10 (double-leg version)	Weeks 11 through 20 (single-leg version)	Page
SB bridge (double leg to single leg)	5 reps, adding 1 rep per week up to 15	5 reps per leg, adding 1 rep per week up to 15	128
SB leg curl (double leg to single leg)	5 reps, adding 1 rep per week up to 15	5 reps per leg, adding 1 rep per week up to 15	129
SB hip lift (double leg to single leg)	5 reps, adding 1 rep per week up to 15	5 reps per leg, adding 1 rep per week up to 15	128

Metabolic Protocols

These advanced protocols, called *metabolic protocols*, are giant sets that provide superior conditioning, strength, power, and power endurance targeted toward one body part. They're great for advanced athletes who are looking to add high-level training to their current training protocol. You can also use them as short training sessions when traveling or when time is tight. Metabolic protocols are a perfect way to finish a hypertrophy or strength workout in order to bring a lot of blood to the body part being worked. Flush sets have always been popular with bodybuilders as a method of finishing a workout.

The metabolic protocols also have given rise to the IHP prefatigue system of endurance training, which allows endurance athletes to cut down on their training volume. For example, use 1 to 5 sets of the JC Leg Crank immediately before a training run so as to prefatigue the legs and make a short training run feel like a much longer run. This approach has yielded incredible results with endurance and combat athletes, reducing the repetitive wear and tear of endurance training while increasing training intensity.

You must establish a base before jumping into metabolic protocols. As a general rule, you must be able to perform 3 sets of each exercise as a workout and not feel sore the next day. Following this training progression allows you to enjoy the training process and avoid being crippled by DOMS the day after abusive training or straining joints that are not ready for advanced training.

This program (tables 7.14 and 7.15) was inspired by industry lead, Vern Gambetta, and provides superior leg training for the intermediate athlete who has a good base of conditioning. It is popular with all athletes who need strong, durable legs and can be used as a leg flush after a leg day, as a quick session during the season, or as preparation for the rigors of preseason training.

THE EXERCISES

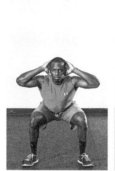 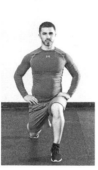 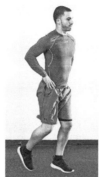 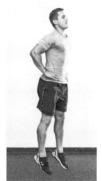

Bodyweight double-leg squat.　Bodyweight alternating lunge.　Alternating split jump.　Squat jump.

THE HOW

TABLE 7.14 JC Leg Crank

Exercise	Reps	Page
Bodyweight double-leg squat	24	42
Bodyweight alternating lunge	12 per leg	43
Alternating split jump	12 per leg	66
Squat jump	12	66

Circuit progression: During weeks 1 and 2, perform the program twice a week (Monday and Friday). During weeks 3 through 6, perform the program once a week. Table 7.15 lists the set progressions and the recovery times for each week.

TABLE 7.15 Weekly Protocol for JC Leg Crank

Week	Sets	Recovery between exercises	Recovery between sets
1	2	45 sec.	2 min.
2	3	30 sec.	90 min.
3	4	15 sec.	60 sec.
4	5	15 sec.	30 sec.
5	5	No recovery	No recovery
6	6	No recovery	No recovery

This program (table 7.16) provides superior back training for the intermediate athlete who has a good base of conditioning, and it is popular with swimmers and throwing athletes. It can be used as a leg flush after a back day, as a quick session during the season, or as preparation for the rigors of preseason training.

THE EXERCISES

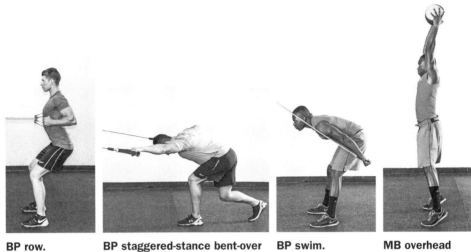

BP row.

BP staggered-stance bent-over alternating row.

BP swim.

MB overhead slam.

THE HOW

TABLE 7.16   JC Meta Back

Perform the exercises in the sequence shown here as a giant set with no rest between exercises. This giant set can be performed up to three times with 1 to 3 minutes of rest between sets. You can perform the JC Meta Back one or two times per week with at least two days of rest between each day.

Exercise	Reps	Page
BP row	20	77
BP staggered-stance bent-over alternating row	10 per arm and leg (20 reps per arm total)	79
BP swim	20	84
MB overhead slam	10	120

Metabolic Chest Training: JC Meta Chest

The JC Meta Chest comes in two versions. The 1.0 is the original version and uses band and bodyweight exercises. The 2.0 version was featured in *Men's Health* as a quick method of developing explosive pushing and punching power as well as improving bench press capability. Both of these protocols (table 7.17 and 7.18) are popular with well-conditioned athletes who need pushing and punching power. They can be used as a chest flush after a chest day, as a quick session during the season, or as a preparatory protocol to get ready for the rigors of preseason training.

Perform the exercises in either program in the sequence shown in the table as a giant set with no rest between exercises. These giant sets can be performed up to three times with 1 to 3 minutes of rest between each set. Some elite athletes have even completed two JC Meta Chest protocols back to back without any rest. You can perform several sets of either JC Meta Chest protocol 1 or 2 times per week with at least two days of rest between each day.

THE EXERCISES

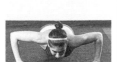

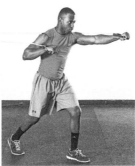

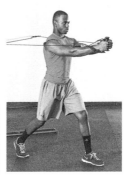

Bodyweight push-up.

BP staggered-stance alternating press.

BP staggered-stance fly.

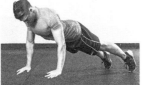

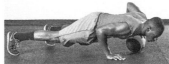

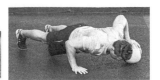

Explosive push-up.

MB single-arm push-off.

MB crossover push-up.

THE HOW

TABLE 7.17 JC Meta Chest 1.0

Exercise	Reps	Page
Bodyweight push-up	20	44
BP staggered-stance alternating press	20 per leg (40 total)	75
BP staggered-stance fly	10 per leg (20 total)	76
Explosive push-up	10	69

TABLE 7.18 JC Meta Chest 2.0

Exercise	Reps	Page
Bodyweight push-up	20	44
MB single-arm push-off	5 per side (10 total)*	114
MB crossover push-up	5 per side (10 total)*	115
Explosive push-up	10	69

*Elite athletes can attempt to perform 10 per side (20 total).

Gary's Dumbbell Matrix

This dumbbell protocol is part of the matrix training system introduced to me by the physical therapist Gary Gray, one of the nicest professionals and human beings I have had the pleasure to call a friend and colleague. I have modified it somewhat, but its main structure stays intact. It's a continuous 72 repetitions involving four stages that invoke all four pillars in three planes of motion. It is composed of a pressing sequence (three exercises), a curling sequence (three exercises), a reaching lunge sequence (three exercises), and a reaching lunge to press sequence (three exercises). You perform 6 reps of each exercise (3 per side), and thus the total circuit is 72 repetitions. Aim to complete the circuit in 1:45 to 2:00 minutes (table 7.19).

Although this program is presented in the metabolic section, you could easily use it as a general fitness protocol or even as a warm-up if you use lighter dumbbells. However, when using aggressive loads (i.e., dumbbells heavier than 10 percent of body weight) and keeping the protocol under 1:45 minutes, the grease can get pretty hot. Heart rates can go higher than 200 bpm when doing multiple sets with short rest periods (under 2 minutes).

Perform the exercises in the sequence as shown. Your goal is to perform the 72 repetitions continuously. To get there, follow this progression:

1. Start with individual exercises, performing 2 or 3 sets of 8 to 16 repetitions per side on different days of the week. Typically a person would spend two or three weeks at this stage to learn and perfect the execution of the exercises.

2. Once you've mastered the individual exercises, rehearse the entire circuit with body weight. This application is a great warm-up. It takes 1:30 to 1:45 minutes; rest 2 or 3 minutes between sets. Perform 3 sets before each workout on three days a week. Stay in this phase for one to three weeks.

3. Once you can easily perform several sets of the complete matrix using body weight, add light dumbbells (about 5 percent of body weight). Go for complete recovery between sets, about 2 minutes. Perform 3 sets on one to three days a week.

4. Progress to using dumbbells that are about 7 percent of body weight, with complete recovery between sets (about 3 minutes per set). Perform 2 or 3 sets on one or two days a week.

5. Progress to using dumbbells that are 10 to 12 percent of body weight, with complete recovery between sets (about 4 minutes per set). Perform 2 or 3 sets on one or two days a week.

The matrix can be part of a weekly routine performed indefinitely with light weight (5 percent body weight). When performing the matrix with heavier loads, periodize the protocol into cycles; for example, four weeks at 5 percent body weight, four weeks at 7 percent body weight, four weeks at 10 percent body weight, and four weeks at 12 percent body weight.

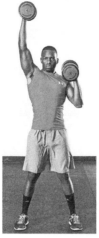
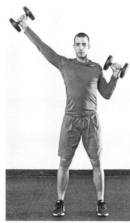
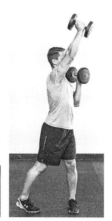

**DB or KB over-
head press.**

**DB or KB overhead Y
press.**

**DB or KB cross
overhead press.**

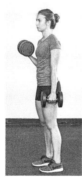
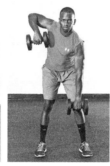
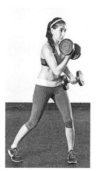

**DB or KB
biceps curl.**

**DB or KB upright
row.**

**DB or KB cross
uppercut.**

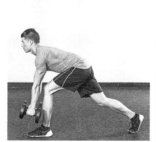
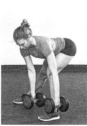
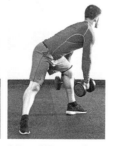

**DB or KB front reaching
lunge.**

**DB or KB lateral
reaching lunge.**

**DB or KB rotating
reaching lunge.**

> continued

THE HOW

TABLE 7.19 Gary's Dumbbell Matrix

Use dumbbells for all exercises.

PRESSING SEQUENCE		
Exercise	**Reps**	**Page**
DB or KB overhead press (alternating)	3 per side	98
DB or KB overhead Y press (alternating)	3 per side	99
DB or KB cross overhead press (alternating)	3 per side	100

CURLING SEQUENCE		
Exercise	**Reps**	**Page**
DB or KB biceps curl (alternating)	3 per side	101
DB or KB upright row (alternating)	3 per side	103
DB or KB cross uppercut (alternating)	3 per side	104

REACHING LUNGE SEQUENCE		
Exercise	**Reps**	**Page**
DB or KB front reaching lunge (alternating)	3 per side	94
DB or KB lateral reaching lunge (alternating)	3 per side	95
DB or KB rotating reaching lunge (alternating)	3 per side	96

REACHING LUNGE TO PRESS SEQUENCE		
Exercise	**Reps**	**Page**
DB or KB front reaching lunge (alternating) and simultaneous DB or KB overhead press	3 per side	94 98
DB or KB lateral reaching lunge (alternating) and simultaneous DB or KB overhead press	3 per side	95 98
DB or KB rotating reaching lunge (alternating) and simultaneous DB or KB overhead press	3 per side	96 98

Conclusion

Functional training is just not a rehabilitation methodology or some light training done for complex neurological reasons. The programs in this chapter show that you can program functional training to teach sound movement patterns, develop high strength levels, and provide power endurance that just won't quit. Additionally, the programs show how easily you can perform functional training in familiar areas, such as fields and hotel rooms, with accessible, inexpensive equipment. The programs provided here are just the beginning of what you can do with the programming ideas and exercises in this book.

Chapter 8 describes the most powerful way to combine functional training and traditional training—the IHP hybrid training system. This system seamlessly integrates traditional strength training and functional training. This is where you'll be able to put the hustle behind the muscle!

CHAPTER 8

Hybrid Programming

No functional training book is complete without a detailed system that combines functional training with other popular and effective training philosophies and systems. Fitness professionals, coaches, and the general public have become increasingly aware of the effectiveness of functional training and other modalities in improving human performance. With all of the information now available, the question that keeps coming up is, "Can we mix modalities or training philosophies to get the best adaptation from the best modalities?" The answer is a resounding *yes*! Although the philosophies of training methods may be in direct opposition, the right approach can combine two different training methods to create a seamless hybrid system. The best example of this hybrid training is combining bodybuilding or traditional strength training with functional training.

Another factor to consider when looking at consolidating training is time. It's often difficult for athletes to get the training they need in a single week. This is especially true with the strength and conditioning portion of training. With all of the technical and academic work demanded of athletes, strength and conditioning workouts are often sacrificed. Working as a personal trainer and coach over the last 20 years, I had to develop training methods that would allow me to address strength, hypertrophy, power, and any performance or rehabilitative concerns within a 30- to 60-minute block of time per day in a couple of hours per week. During this time I successfully created hybrid programs that combine traditional strength methods and the latest developments in functional training. What follows are the results of those 20 years of research and development: the IHP Hybrid Training System

This hybrid system combines the best of functional training and the best of traditional hypertrophy, strength, and power training. Each training approach has excellent attributes, and all athletes want to capitalize on the best practices to obtain optimal results. After reviewing my clients' training charts for months, I saw a pattern in what was happening in my practice, and a system of integration emerged. I named that system of integration the *Three-Tier Integration System (3TIS)*. The 3TIS has been the foundation of the IHP Hybrid Training System, and its development is a major ingredient in IHP's success.

Three-Tier Integration System

In the 3TIS, modalities that were once mutually exclusive coexist in one training program. Not only does the 3TIS allow the athlete to work on a muscle, it also allows the athlete to work on muscle systems and, more importantly, the hustle behind the muscle.

The 3TIS is so named because we have three ways to integrate a functional modality (or exercise) into a traditional workout:

1. We can introduce the modality into the warm-up or cool-down of the workout.
2. We can use the modality to build up to a specific body part.
3. We can use the modality to unload a body part from traditional work.

Let's assume you need standard hypertrophy and strength training. You also see the value of functional training. How can we mix these training approaches into one session? Let's go through each level of integration in more detail to answer that question.

Warm-Up and Cool-Down

Any of the functional modalities or exercises in this book can be incorporated into the warm-up of any training session. This is called the *general warm-up* approach. The general warm-up is usually a total-body routine that uses any modality you like. An example of a general warm-up is the Chopper program in chapter 7. This is a great way to introduce functional training to someone who is stuck in the traditional training paradigm.

The warm-up approach to integration can also be extended to a specific warm-up in preparation for traditional isolation training. You can functionally warm up a body part before training it traditionally. For example, anterior reaches make a great warm-up for lunges or squats. You can also include them at the end of the workout to provide the balance and stability missing from many traditional exercises, such as leg extensions and leg curls.

Band or cable pushing and pulling exercises can prepare the body for traditional pressing or pulling exercises (e.g., bench press, cable row). Bands and pulleys allow you to use a standing position, which provides greater functional carryover and core training compared with machine-based upper-body training.

The eclectic training approaches used in the warm-up level of integration will not feel like a threat or even a change to anyone set on traditional training; the traditional component of the training goes unchanged. Although conditioning professionals recognize the enormous role of a warm-up, most athletes don't consider the warm-up or cool-down to be part of the training session. For this reason, they may readily try a new training approach during these times. The effectiveness of these 10 to 15 minutes of the workout can certainly compare to the 15 minutes of treatment experienced in an aggressive therapy session. And of course, 10 to 15 minutes three or four times per week can end up totaling 45 to 60 minutes. I have seen enormous improvements in stability and power output in this amount of time. This application of functional training has played a major role in the performance gains of my athletes.

Build-Up

Once the functional training philosophy has been fully adopted, it's time to get a little more aggressive using the build-up tier of integration. A build-up is an aggressive, specific warm-up. It uses 2 or 3 sets of increasing intensity to prepare the athlete for the target training load. Many traditional resistance training exercises can start with a more functional position during the lighter sets (e.g., standing instead of sitting). When the unstable environment of the functional position prevents the athlete from performing the exercise with good form, she can complete a few more supported sets to work on absolute strength and hypertrophy. This method of integration is similar to the pre-exhaust and pyramid loading methods popularized in the 1960s and 1970s. Here are some examples of the build-up:

1. **Bent-over rows, unstable to stable.** Bent-over rows can be performed in a freestanding manner (i.e., staggered and single-leg stances) until the weight is so heavy that the hips and lower back can't support the exercise in good form. Go to technical failure, not physiological failure. After reaching a point of technical failure, go to supported bent-over rows (i.e., hand on a bench) or cable rows.

2. **Single-leg squats to leg presses.** Perform several sets of single-leg squats with incremental loads (i.e., increase range of motion or add load with medicine ball or dumbbells) until you can't perform any more with good form. Then go to a single- or double-leg press for heavy, stable work.

Unload

The unloading method is the most popular level of integration in my hybrid system. In this tier, the prime movers are targeted for traditional heavy hypertrophy or strength on one day of the week and are unloaded with functional training on the other days of the week. Although the prime movers may not get traditional heavy work on the unloading day, the neurological demand of functional exercises still maintains a high intensity and volume. Here is an example of how the unloading level of integration works.

Let's say that you have a heavy leg and hip day scheduled for Monday, a heavy push day for Wednesday, and a heavy pulling day for Friday. On Monday, you work the legs and hips with traditional training (e.g., squats, lunges, deadlifts) and unload the pushing and pulling muscles with functional modalities (e.g., stability ball push-ups, band pulls). On Wednesday, you focus on the push muscles with traditional training (e.g., incline bench press, flat bench press, dips) and unload the legs and hips and the pull muscles with functional modalities (e.g., lateral reaching lunges, recline pulls). On Friday, you target the pull muscles with traditional training (e.g., pull-downs, cable rows, upright rows) and unload the legs and hips and the push muscles with functional modalities (e.g., anterior reaches, band presses). Each day, you throw in a little rotation work or other specialized therapy work.

The order and scheme used in this level of integration can vary. One method is to perform all of the traditional exercises first and then finish with the functional exercises. Table 8.1 illustrates what this workout might look like.

TABLE 8.1   Sample Unloading Scheme With Traditional Exercises First

MONDAY

Exercise	Sets and reps
Barbell squat	3 × 10
DB or KB lunge	3 × 10
Barbell deadlift	3 × 10
SB hands-on-ball push-up	3 × 10
BP row	3 × 10
BP short rotation (10 to 2 o'clock)	3 × 10

WEDNESDAY

Exercise	Sets and reps
Barbell incline bench press	3 × 10
Barbell flat bench press	3 × 10
Dip (load as needed)	3 × 10
Single-leg squat	3 × 10
BP staggered-stance CLA row	3 × 10
SB skier	3 × 10

FRIDAY

Exercise	Sets and reps
Pull-down	3 × 10
BP row	3 × 10
Barbell upright row	3 × 10
Single-leg CLA anterior reach	3 × 10
BP staggered-stance CLA press	3 × 10
BP high-to-low chop	3 × 10

Another scheme that can be used to unload is the IHP hybrid complex scheme. This scheme uses circuits with traditional and functional training modalities. The circuits can be made of two exercises: a traditional exercise and a functional exercise (i.e., biplex), a traditional exercise and two functional exercises (i.e., triplex), or a traditional exercise and three functional exercises (i.e., quadplex). Table 8.2 illustrates what the workout in table 8.1 would look like using biplexes to integrate the strength and hypertrophy of traditional training with the movement skill of the functional modality.

Hybrid Complexes

The 3TIS was my first attempt to combine diverse systems of training into a single workout. As previously mentioned, the unloading level of integration was the most significant development; it is the most popular and powerful method of integration. This section explains the methodology used to create complexes that integrate and unload one body part with functional training while isolating and loading another body part with traditional strength training.

TABLE 8.2 Sample Unloading Scheme Using Hybrid Biplexes

MONDAY

Exercise	Sets and reps
Barbell squat	3 × 10
SB hands-on-ball push-up	3 × 10
DB or KB lunge	3 × 10
BP row	3 × 10
Barbell deadlift	3 × 10
BP short rotation (10 to 2 o'clock)	3 × 10

WEDNESDAY

Exercise	Sets and reps
Barbell incline bench press	3 × 10
Single-leg squat	3 × 10
Barbell flat bench press	3 × 10
BP staggered-stance CLA row	3 × 10
Dip (load as needed)	3 × 10
SB skier	3 × 10

FRIDAY

Exercise	Sets and reps
Pull-down	3 × 10
Single-leg CLA anterior reach	3 × 10
BP row	3 × 10
BP staggered-stance CLA press	3 × 10
Barbell upright row	3 × 10
BP high-to-low chop	3 × 10

The IHP Hybrid Training System is a complex of exercises that target specific components of performance. Complexes combine traditional exercises (to provide strength and hypertrophy) with functional exercises (to hit the body in a different manner than traditional training). The functional and rehabilitative exercises usually tackle components that traditional exercises miss, such as engaging various planes of motion, using various levers, moving through various ranges of motion, and engaging stabilizers and neutralizers in various capacities. Hybrid complexes scheme can contain two (biplex), three (triplex), or four (quadplex) exercises.

Biplexes

In biplexes, the first exercise is a primary exercise that focuses on the major physiological quality of interest. For example, if we are trying to increase lean muscle mass in the lower body, we use a hypertrophy leg exercise such as the squat or leg press for the first exercise. The next exercise is usually a core exercise that is driven by another body part and action (e.g., a push or pull), therefore unloading that body part. An example of an exercise that uses a pushing movement to drive the core but unload the chest is the SB hands-on-ball push-up. This exercise does not tax the chest and offers some active recovery from bench-pressing days, which is why it is called an *unloading exercise*. These two exercises would constitute the biplex:

1. Barbell squat or machine leg press
2. SB hands-on-ball push-up

If an entire program consisted of biplexes, it would be 50 percent traditional hypertrophy training and 50 percent functional training, excluding the warm-up. Biplexes are excellent for athletes who want to focus on gaining muscle while still addressing other performance and rehabilitative concerns such as core stability. Here are some more sample biplexes and the rationale behind them.

Biplex 1

1. Traditional leg exercise: machine leg press
2. Unloading chest and core: BP staggered-stance CLA press

Reasoning: Provide the legs and hips with a strength and hypertrophy stimulus. Unload the chest with a core exercise that lengthens and strengthens the hip flexors.

Biplex 2

1. Traditional chest exercise: barbell flat bench press
2. Unloading legs and hips: single-leg CLA anterior reach

Reasoning: Provide the chest with a strength and hypertrophy stimulus. Address lower-body rehabilitative concerns (i.e., hip, knee, and ankle stability) during the rest period.

Biplex 3

1. Traditional back exercise: pull-down
2. Rotational core: BP short rotation (10 to 2 o'clock)

Reasoning: Provide the back with a strength and hypertrophy stimulus. Address total-body and core stiffness rotational strength and stability.

Triplexes

To add more functional training to a biplex, we can add a third exercise. Assuming we are focusing on the legs with the traditional training and unloading the chest with the SB hand-on-ball push-up, we might choose a functional pulling exercise such as a BP staggered-stance CLA row for the third exercise. The BP staggered-stance CLA row trains the posterior muscles of the core and enhances flexibility in the hip flexors. The triplex hybrid complex would look like this:

1. Barbell squat or machine leg press
2. SB hands-on-ball push-up
3. BP staggered-stance CLA row

The triplex splits the training emphasis to favor functional training: approximately 67 percent functional and 33 percent hypertrophy, excluding the warm-up and cool-down. This is my preferred format for clients who have developed a high-intensity training base and can go through this circuit without fading in the traditional lifts. Here are a few more examples of triplexes and the rationale behind them.

Triplex 1

1. Traditional leg exercise: barbell squat
2. Unloading chest and core: side T plank
3. Unloading back and core: BP row

Reasoning: Provide the extensors of the legs and hips with strength and hypertrophy stimulus. Unload the chest and shoulders with a core exercise that strengthens the lateral aspect of the core. Unload the back muscles with a basic exercise that improves shoulder stability and postural mechanics.

Triplex 2

1. Traditional chest exercise: barbell incline bench press
2. Unloading legs, hips, and core: DB or KB lateral reaching lunge
3. Rotational core: BP high-to-low chop

Reasoning: Provide the chest with a strength and hypertrophy stimulus. Unload the legs and hips, address lower-body and core stability, and address triplanar range of motion. Train rotational strength and stability.

Triplex 3

1. Traditional back exercise: pull-down
2. Unloading chest and core: BP staggered-stance CLA press
3. Unloading legs, hips, and balance: single-leg CLA anterior reach

Reasoning: Provide the back with a strength and hypertrophy stimulus. Unload the chest and train total-core and shoulder (scapula) stability. Functionally unload lower-body balance and stability.

Quadplexes

Many endurance athletes do not need to increase muscle mass, but they do want to be stronger and not lose any of the muscle mass they have. For these athletes, we can consider adding a fourth exercise to the triplex, making it a quadplex. The fourth exercise can deal with any other training concern. For example, let's consider a soccer player who has had problems with lower abdominal weakness and groin pain. The fourth exercise can address this deficiency. The X-up would make a great choice for the fourth exercise in this complex. The quadplex thus looks like this:

1. Barbell squat or machine leg press
2. SB hands-on-ball push-up
3. BP staggered-stance CLA row
4. X-up

Of all the complexes, the quadplex provides the greatest amount of functional training—75 percent functional and 25 percent traditional, not counting the warm-up and cool-down. This is a popular approach during the power-endurance phase of periodization and with endurance athletes who do not require significant hypertrophy. Here are a few examples of quadplexes and the rationale behind them.

Quadplex 1

1. Traditional leg exercise: barbell deadlift
2. Unloading chest and core: SB hands-on-ball push-up
3. Unloading back and core: recline pull (row)
4. Rotational core: SB skier

Reasoning: Provide the legs and hips with a strength and hypertrophy stimulus. Unload the chest with a core exercise that lengthens and strengthens the hip flexors. Unload the back while training hip and back extensor strength and lengthening the front core. Train rotational strength and range of motion.

Quadplex 2

1. Traditional shoulder exercise: barbell overhead press
2. Unloading legs and core: MB ABC squat
3. Unloading flexibility and core: SB rollout
4. Rotational core: BP high-to-low chop

Reasoning: Provide the shoulders with a strength and hypertrophy stimulus. Unload the legs and hips and address lower-body stability and triplanar range of motion. Unload the pulling muscles while lengthening and strengthening the anterior core. Address core stiffness and rotational stability.

Quadplex 3

1. Traditional back exercise: dumbbell bent-over row
2. Unloading chest and core: BP staggered-stance fly
3. Unloading leg and core: MB lunge with rotation
4. Rotational core: SB skier

Reasoning: Provide the back with a strength and hypertrophy stimulus. Unload the chest and train anterior hip flexibility and stability. Unload the legs and hips and address lower-body balance and triplanar stability.

Execution of Complexes

The sets and repetitions for the hybrid complexes are easy to assign. The first exercise in a hybrid is a traditional exercise and follows the standard repetition scheme described in most periodization models. For example, during a hypertrophy cycle you would perform the first exercise in a hybrid complex for 8 to 15 repetitions, and during a strength cycle you would perform the first exercise for 4 to 6 repetitions. During each phase, you perform all functional exercises for 10 to 20 repetitions per side or for 10 to 20 seconds for balance or isometric exercises. This is how triplex 3 would look during a hypertrophy phase:

1. Traditional back exercise: pull-down (8-15 reps)
2. Unloading chest and core: BP staggered-stance CLA press (10-20 reps per right and left stance)

3. Unloading legs, hips, and balance: single-leg CLA anterior reach (10-20 reps per right and left leg)

The same triplex would look like this during a strength phase:

1. Traditional back exercise: pull-down (4-6 reps)
2. Unloading chest and core: BP staggered-stance CLA press (10-20 reps per right and left stance)
3. Unloading legs, hips, and balance: single-leg CLA anterior reach (10-20 reps per right and left leg)

During the power and power-endurance cycles, we pair a traditional strength exercise with an explosive equivalent and perform both for 5 repetitions. During the power cycle, we rest 60 seconds between the traditional exercise and the explosive equivalent. During the power-endurance cycle, we eliminate the rest period between the traditional exercise and the explosive equivalent. All unloading functional exercises continue to be performed for 10 to 20 repetitions per limb or for 10 to 20 seconds for balance and isometric exercises.

This is how triplex 3 would look during a power phase:

1. Traditional back exercise: pull-down (5 reps)
2. 60-second rest
3. Back explosive equivalent: MB overhead slam (5 reps)
4. Unloading legs, hips, and balance: single-leg CLA anterior reach (10 to 20 reps per right and left leg)

This is what triplex 3 would look like during a power-endurance phase:

1. Traditional back exercise: pull-down (5 reps)
2. No rest
3. Back explosive equivalent: MB overhead slam (5 reps)
4. Unloading legs, hips, and balance: single-leg CLA anterior reach (10-20 reps per right and left leg)

When training with the IHP hybrids, the athlete moves continuously. However, this does not mean she races through a workout. The workout can move along at a deliberate tempo: 20 to 30 seconds for each exercise, 15 to 20 seconds to transition between exercises, and 30 to 60 seconds between circuits. Expand the rest periods if the quality of the work is diminishing. Also, you can tailor the tempo to the goal of the cycle. For example, in a strength cycle the athlete may want to take longer rest periods than in a power-endurance cycle.

The IHP Hybrid Training System is excellent for large groups. It keeps everyone busy, and everyone gets the most out of the training time. A three-exercise complex designed around a lifting rack can keep four athletes productive with no downtime, with one athlete squatting, one spotting (on deck, resting), one performing band rotations (attach the band to the lifting rack), and one doing rotational push-ups for shoulder stability.

The hybrid training system is extremely flexible; it can combine every modality you can think of, from stretching protocols to speed, agility, and quickness drills. The hybrid circuits should be simple and easy to execute; they should not become a circus act! Remember, coordination, dynamic balance, and stability are fast to develop because their enhancement is a neural event. Control and stability are sequencing (i.e., neural) issues, not hypertrophy issues. It takes some practice but uses little energy once mastered, just like riding a bike. Now, let's take a look at some more examples of hybrid programming and additional hybrid programming principles.

Periodizing and Programming Hybrid Programs

Periodization of the hybrid program follows the same model discussed in chapter 6. Here is a review of the phases (or cycles) and the volume associated with each phase. See table 8.3 for a summary.

Conditioning and Hypertrophy

A high volume of work with a moderate intensity or load characterizes this cycle. The cycle length is approximately four weeks and the hybrid complexes are performed for enough sets so that each body part gets 12 to 20 sets per week with 8 to 15 repetitions per set for the traditional exercises. For example, if you are performing three triplexes on a leg day, do 3 to 5 sets of each triplex so that the traditional exercises total 9 to 15 sets per week. Although the lower range of 9 sets is not within the range of 12 to 20 sets per week, it still offers significant training. The standard goal for the set range for three triplexes is 4 sets each (12 sets per week).

Strength

The strength phase is characterized by low-volume, high-intensity training. The cycle length is approximately four weeks and the hybrid complexes are performed for enough sets so that each body part gets 10 to 12 sets per week with 4 to 6 repetitions per set for the traditional exercises. As in the hypertrophy cycle, if you are performing three triplexes on a chest day, do 3 or 4 sets of each triplex so that the traditional exercises total 9 to 12 sets per week. Although the lower range of 9 sets is not within the range of 10 to 12 sets per week, it is basically equivalent as far as training is concerned. You can easily perform 12 sets per week by performing 4 sets of three triplexes.

TABLE 8.3 Periodization of Hybrid Training

Cycle	Cycle length	Sets per week per body part	Reps of traditional exercise	Reps of functional/ unloading exercise
Conditioning and hypertrophy	4 weeks	12 to 20	8 to 15	10 to 20 reps or sec.
Strength	4 weeks	10 to 12	4 to 6	10 to 20 reps or sec.
Power	4 weeks	8 to 12	5 and 5 (rest 60 sec. between exercises)	10 to 20 reps or sec.
Power endurance	4 weeks	8 to 12	5 and 5 (no rest)	10 to 20 reps or sec.

Power

The power phase is characterized by low-volume, high-speed training. The cycle length is approximately four weeks and the hybrid complexes are performed for enough sets so that each body part gets 8 to 12 sets that consist of 5 repetitions of a strength exercise and 5 repetitions of an explosive equivalent exercise, with 60 seconds of rest between the first and second exercise in the power complex. For example, if you are performing three triplexes on a back day, do 3 or 4 sets of each triplex so that the traditional back strength and explosive equivalent combination totals 9 to 12 sets per week, well within the 8 to 12 range.

Power Endurance

The power-endurance cycle is identical to the power cycle except for the rest period between the first and second exercises of the power complex. During the power-endurance cycle, there is no rest period between the traditional strength exercise and the explosive equivalent. Performing three triplexes on a chest day, do three or four sets of each triplex so that the traditional chest strength and explosive equivalent combination totals 9 to 12 sets per week. This falls within our 8 to 12 sets weekly range.

Sample Programs

For many athletes, getting bigger and stronger is definitely on the to-do list. The hybrid model is an efficient way to meet this goal. Table 8.4 illustrates the general approach to designing a monthly hybrid that combines strength and

TABLE 8.4 Sample IHP Hybrid Conditioning and Hypertrophy or Strength Template

Day 1 Legs and hips	Day 2 Push	Day 3 Pull
TS leg exercise (parallel stance) FT unloading push exercise FT upper-body ROM/rehab exercise	TS push exercise (incline) FT unloading leg/hip exercise FT lower-body balance/ ROM exercise	TS pull exercise (downward pull) FT unloading leg/hip exercise FT vibration or rehab exercise
TS leg exercise (staggered-stance alternating) FT unloading pull exercise FT rotation exercise (side to side)	TS push exercise (straight) FT unloading pull exercise FT rotation exercise (low to high)	TS pull exercise (inward pull) FT unloading push exercise FT rotation exercise (high to low)
TS leg exercise (hip dominant) FT unloading push–pull exercise FT front core exercise	TS push exercise (decline) FT unloading leg/hip pull exercise FT back core exercise	TS pull exercise (upward pull) FT unloading leg/hip push exercise FT back core exercise

TS: traditional strength, FT: functional training, ROM: range of motion function. This template shows the category of each exercise so that plugging in exercises within the same category can yield an unlimited number of programs. Remember, this is just one of many templates; your imagination is the only limit to programming in the IHP hybrid training system.

The set and repetition ranges for the hybrid conditioning and hypertrophy or strength template are as follows:

Conditioning and hypertrophy cycle: 3 or 5 sets of each triplex, with 8 to 15 repetitions of the traditional exercise and 10 to 20 repetitions or seconds (if isometric or balance) of the functional training exercises

Strength cycle: 3 or 4 sets of each triplex, with 4 to 6 repetitions of the traditional exercise and 10 to 20 repetitions or seconds (if isometric or balance) of the functional training exercises

Plugging in some of the exercises from this book yields the comprehensive hybrid program shown in table 8.5. If each triplex is performed for approximately 4 sets, each body part gets about 12 sets per week. During a conditioning and hypertrophy cycle, the first exercise (i.e., the traditional exercise) would be performed for 8 to 15 repetitions, and for a strength cycle the first exercise would be performed for 4 to 6 repetitions.

The tempo of the strength training exercises need not be slow. Although you can use slower tempos, especially for traditional strength training, I prefer the standard tempo of 1 to 2 seconds per repetition for all exercises during the hypertrophy and strength phases. The rest between exercises depends on the intensity of the exercise. A slow 15- to 30-second walk from station to station is usually enough recovery to allow the athlete to continue with good form and intensity. The rest period between triplexes (i.e., the third and first exercises of a triplex) can range from 1 to 2 minutes, again depending on how heavy the training load is for the traditional and functional exercises. After completing a triplex for 3 or 4 sets, you can take a 2- to 5-minute rest to set up the next triplex and mentally prepare for a high-intensity output.

TABLE 8.5 Sample IHP Hybrid Conditioning and Hypertrophy or Strength Workout

Day 1 Legs and hips	Day 2 Push	Day 3 Pull
Barbell squat BP staggered-stance alternating press SB rollout	Barbell incline bench press DB or KB lateral reaching lunge Single-leg CLA anterior reach	Pull-down DB or KB front reaching lunge Vibration blade 12 o'clock oscillation
DB or KB lunge Recline pull (row) BP short rotation (10 to 2 o'clock)	Barbell flat bench press BP staggered-stance CLA compound row BP low-to-high chop	Seated cable row T push-up BP high-to-low chop
Barbell deadlift BP push–pull SB knee tuck	Dip (load as needed) BP staggered-stance (or single-leg) alternating row 45-degree back extension	Barbell upright row BP staggered-stance (or single-leg) alternating press SB reverse hyperextension

We can follow the same model for the power and power-endurance cycles as we did for the hypertrophy and strength cycles. Table 8.6 shows a template for the power and power-endurance cycles. Simply use any of the exercises that match the category in the template to create a monthly power or power-endurance workout.

The repetition range for the power and power-endurance template is as follows:

Power cycle: 3 or 4 sets of each triplex, with 5 reps of the traditional exercise and explosive exercise with a 1-minute rest between exercises, resting about 30 seconds before going on to 10 to 20 reps of the third functional training exercise

Power-endurance cycle: 3 to 4 sets of each triplex, with 5 reps of the traditional and explosive exercises with no rest between exercises, resting about 30 seconds before going on to 10 to 20 reps of the third functional training exercise

Plugging in some of the exercises from previous chapters yields the program in table 8.7. This is just one of the many power and power-endurance workouts that can be designed using the triplex template from table 8.6. Again, the only difference between the power and the power-endurance cycles is the rest period between the first (traditional) exercise and the second (explosive equivalent) exercise. The athlete rests 1 minute between exercises during the power cycle and doesn't rest during the power-endurance cycle.

The focus during the power and power-endurance phases is speed of movement. The first exercise in each triplex is performed with a load that is heavy enough to maintain strength but light enough to allow the athlete to move the weight in a dynamic fashion. Normally I advise a load that allows about 8 repetitions when performing the 5 heavy repetitions needed in the power phase. These 5 repetitions need to be performed at good speed with excellent form when lifting the weight (control the descent), allowing a nice combination of load and speed during the strength exercise. The explosive exercise should be a simple exercise that allows an all-out effort with excellent speed.

During the power cycle, the rest between the first and second exercises is approximately 1 minute. Efforts on the explosive equivalent must be personal-record

TABLE 8.6 Sample IHP Hybrid Power or Power-Endurance Template

Day 1 Legs and hips	Day 2 Push	Day 3 Pull
TS leg exercise (parallel stance) Explosive leg exercise FT upper-body ROM/rehab exercise	TS push exercise (incline) Explosive push exercise FT lower-body balance/ ROM exercise	TS pull exercise (downward pull) Explosive pull exercise FT vibration or rehab exercise
TS leg exercise (staggered- stance alternating) Explosive leg exercise FT rotation exercise	TS push exercise (straight) Explosive push exercise FT rotation exercise	TS pull exercise (inward pull) Explosive pull exercise FT rotation exercise
TS leg exercise (hip dominant) Explosive leg exercise FT front core exercise	TS push exercise (decline) Explosive push exercise FT back core exercise	TS pull exercise (upward pull) Explosive pull exercise FT back core exercise

TS: traditional strength, FT: functional training, ROM: range of motion

TABLE 8.7 Sample IHP Hybrid Power and Power-Endurance Workout

Day 1 Legs and hips	Day 2 Push	Day 3 Pull
Barbell squat Squat jump SB rollout	Barbell incline bench press MB staggered-stance CLA incline chest throw Single-leg CLA anterior reach	Pull-down MB overhead slam Vibration blade 12 o'clock oscillation
DB or KB lunge Alternating split jump BP short rotation (10 to 2 o'clock)	Barbell flat bench press MB staggered-stance CLA straight chest throw BP low-to-high chop	BP row MB overhead side-to-side slam BP high-to-low chop
Barbell deadlift Burpee SB knee tuck	Dip (load as needed) MB staggered stance CLA decline chest throw 45-degree back extension	Barbell upright row MB reverse scoop throw SB reverse hyperextension

attempts. This can't be emphasized enough. All too often athletes perform the explosive repetitions without game intensity. Take your time and explode, resting your body and mind after each repetition. After completing all power repetitions, slowly walk to the third functional exercise and execute it for 10 to 20 repetitions. Rest 1 to 2 minutes and return to the traditional exercise of the power complex. Rest 3 to 5 minutes between the first, second, and third triplexes.

During the power-endurance cycle, there is no rest between the first and second exercises. Due to the lack of rest, the repetitions are a bit slower than during the power cycle; however, you make an all-out attempt to keep each repetition at a maximum. For endurance sports, you can experiment with higher repetition ranges during power exercises depending on the training volume used for that specific sport. I have used 10 to 15 repetitions with cross country runners with good success. After completing all power repetitions, slowly walk to the third functional exercise and execute it for 10 to 20 repetitions. Rest 1 to 2 minutes and return to the traditional exercise of the power complex. Rest 3 to 5 minutes between the first, second, and third triplexes. However, you may reduce the rest periods between triplexes to create a fast-paced circuit if you would like to add a conditioning element to the hybrid strength training. Running through a triplex three to four times without rest can become challenging from a neurological and metabolic perspective. Now, imagine doing that with three triplexes within a single workout well under 60 minutes, including warm-up and cool-down!

Conclusion

Functional training does not operate in a vacuum, and it does not have to exclude other training modalities, methods, or systems. The hybrid system created at IHP seamlessly combines functional training with any other training system on the planet, from yoga to powerlifting. This hybrid approach has allowed us to create monster athletes and change the face of best practices in fitness.

The final chapter brings it all together and offers the most comprehensive selection of sport-specific functional training ever assembled in a single text. You are in for a real treat!

CHAPTER 9

Sport-Specific Programs

The sport-specific programs in this chapter take the functional exercises related to the four pillars and group them into the best programs. Many of the exercises listed in one program can greatly benefit athletes in other sports. It also worth mentioning that a sport may have three or more distinct positions, each with its own physical build and performance characteristics. For example, a receiver in American football may have more of a soccer profile, but an offensive lineman may have more of a combative profile. Therefore, don't be afraid to mix and match program sections (e.g., triplexes, warm-ups, and core programs).

You can also use the grab-and-go and express protocols from chapter 7 to add specific training for attributes you want to emphasize during your practice, warm-up, cool-down, or homework. For example, athletes can perform the Running Speed-Demon Protocol and the Triple Threat (chapter 7) during commercials while watching TV in the evening. The flexibility and compartmentalization of training units (e.g., express programs, hybrid complexes, metabolic protocols) allow the athlete and coach to start with one of the sample programs and tailor it to the specific sport and athlete.

Unless otherwise specified, the following programs can be performed one to three times per week, depending on the athlete's volume of work and her training experience and maturity (i.e., training base). This is especially true of the power-endurance phase where the hard metabolic training takes place. If an athlete has a heavy competition schedule, she may only be able to do one day per week. Under regular circumstances, two days per week is the norm. If the athlete's schedule is on the lighter side, three days per week can be attempted, but the athlete should be monitored for overtraining symptoms.

High-power arena sports, such as American football and field and ice hockey, require quick bursts of action, lateral changes in direction, and extraordinary physical contact. Running distances rarely cover more than 10 to 20 yards (9-18 m) in a straight line. Quick and short changes of direction are needed during play and are often associated with obstacle avoidance. Because high power acceleration is needed, the posterior chain must be developed to a high level.

Warm-Up for All Workouts

Chopper: 2 to 3 × 10

Single-leg CLA anterior reach: 2 to 3 × 10 to 20 per leg

CONDITIONING

Perform each triplex in order and then start the sequence again. Complete as many sets as indicated. Rest adequately between each exercise to maintain good form and quality of movement, eventually targeting a 30- to 60-second rest period after each exercise. Use enough load to make the assigned repetitions challenging while maintaining good form. Unless otherwise specified, use the progression in table 9.1.

THE EXERCISES

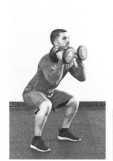

DB or KB squat.

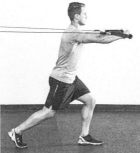

BP staggered-stance press.

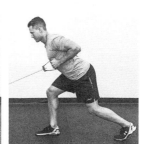

BP staggered-stance CLA low-to-high row.

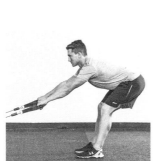

BP deadlift.

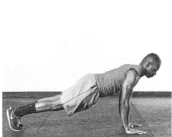

Plank.

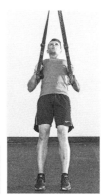

Recline pull (row).

THE HOW

If your fitness level is high, you can start with any week that feels comfortable and repeat the week as many times as necessary to create a strong base of training.

TABLE 9.1 High-Power Intermittent Sports: Conditioning Triplexes

Exercise	Week 1	Week 2	Week 3	Week 4	Page
Triplex 1 1. DB or KB squat 2. BP staggered-stance press 3. BP staggered-stance CLA low-to-high row	2 × 10	3 × 10	3 × 15	4 × 10 to 15	90 74 82
Triplex 2 1. BP deadlift 2. Plank (progress to three-point version) 3. Recline pull (row)	2 × 10	3 × 10	3 × 15	4 × 10 to 15	70 57 46

Core 1

Triple Threat (weeks 1-5)

Slide running: 2 or 3 × 10 to 20 per side

STRENGTH

Perform each triplex in order for the number of sets indicated. Rest adequately between each exercise to maintain good form and quality of movement, eventually targeting a 30- to 60-second rest period after each exercise. Use enough load to make the assigned repetitions challenging while keeping good form. Unless otherwise specified, use the progression in table 9.2.

THE EXERCISES

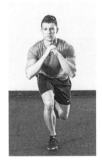
Single-leg squat.

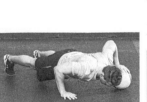
MB crossover push-up.

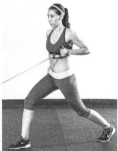
BP staggered-stance CLA compound row.

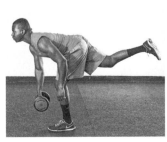
DB or KB single-leg RDL.

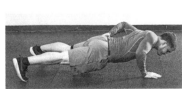
Single-arm eccentrics.

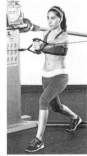
BP push–pull.

> continued

THE HOW

If your fitness level is high, you can start with any week that feels comfortable and repeat the week as many times as necessary to create a strong base of training.

TABLE 9.2 High-Power Intermittent Sports: Strength Triplexes

All single-leg or single-arm exercises should be performed on each leg or arm.

Exercise	Week 1	Week 2	Week 3	Week 4	Page
Triplex 1 1. Single-leg squat (add dumbbells or a medicine ball if necessary) 2. MB crossover push-up 3. BP staggered-stance CLA compound row	1 × 6	2 × 6	3 × 4 to 6	4 × 4 to 6	40 115 83
Triplex 2 1. DB or KB single-leg RDL 2. Single-arm eccentrics 3. BP push–pull	1 × 6	2 × 6	3 × 4 to 6	4 × 4 to 6	92 59 89

Core 2

Triple Threat (weeks 6-10)

Slide running: 2 or 3 × 10 to 20 per side

POWER AND POWER ENDURANCE

Perform each biplex in order for the number of sets indicated. For power, rest 1 minute between the first and second exercises, and then rest 1 to 2 minutes between the second and first exercises. For power endurance, do not rest between the first and second exercises, and then rest 1 minute between the second and first exercises. Use enough load to make the assigned repetitions challenging while maintaining good form. Unless otherwise specified, use the progression in table 9.3.

Additional Warm-Up for Power and Power-Endurance Workouts

Agility ladder split step: 2 or 3 sets

Agility ladder lateral rotational jump: 2 or 3 sets

THE EXERCISES

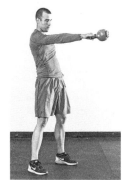

KB single-arm swing.

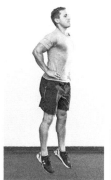

Squat jump.

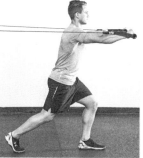

BP staggered-stance press.

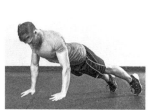

Explosive push-up.

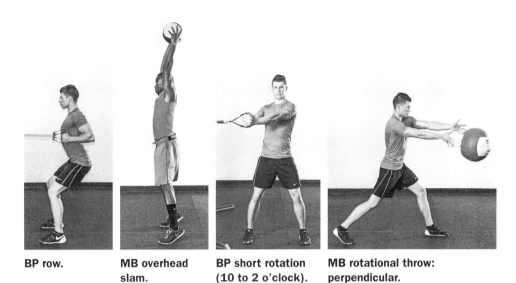

| BP row. | MB overhead slam. | BP short rotation (10 to 2 o'clock). | MB rotational throw: perpendicular. |

THE HOW

If your fitness level is high, you can start with any week that feels comfortable and repeat the week as many times as necessary to create a strong base of training.

TABLE 9.3 High-Power Intermittent Sports: Power and Power-Endurance Biplexes

The single-arm swing should be performed on each arm.

Exercise	Week 1	Week 2	Week 3	Week 4	Page
Biplex 1 1. KB single-arm swing 2. Squat jump	2 × 5 + 5	3 × 5 + 5	3 × 5 + 5	4 × 5 + 5	91 66
Biplex 2 1. BP staggered-stance press 2. Explosive push-up	2 × 5 + 5	3 × 5 + 5	3 × 5 + 5	4 × 5 + 5	74 69
Biplex 3 1. BP row 2. MB overhead slam	2 × 5 + 5	3 × 5 + 5	3 × 5 + 5	4 × 5 + 5	77 120
Biplex 4 1. BP short rotation (10 to 2 o'clock) 2. MB rotational throw: perpendicular	2 × 5 + 5	3 × 5 + 5	3 × 5 + 5	4 × 5 + 5	87 121

5 + 5 indicates 60 seconds of rest between the first and second exercise for power. For power endurance, go straight from the first exercise to the second without resting.

Core 3

For power: Triple Threat (weeks 11-15), slide running (2 or 3 × 10-20 per side)

For power endurance: Triple Threat (weeks 16-20), slide running (3 or 4 × 10-20 per side)

Metabolic

For power: 300-yard (274 m) shuttle (25 yd [22.8 m] × 12), 2 sets, 3 times per week (1:3 work:rest ratio)

For power endurance: 300-yard (274 m) shuttle, 3 or 4 sets, 2 or 3 times per week (1:2 to 1:1 work:rest ratio)

Racket sports such as tennis, badminton, racquetball, and squash have much in common. Players use low positions to get to low balls and overhead positions for serves or smashes. Quick and short changes of directions, especially lateral changes of direction, are needed during 5 to 8 seconds of play. The posterior musculature is especially important due to the low positions and changes of directions.

Warm-Up for All Workouts

Gary's Dumbbell Matrix: 2 sets

CONDITIONING

Perform each triplex in order and then start the sequence again. Complete as many sets as indicated. Rest adequately between each exercise to maintain good form and quality of movement, eventually targeting a 30- to 60-second rest period after each exercise. Use enough load to make the assigned repetitions challenging while maintaining good form. Unless otherwise specified, use the progression in table 9.4.

THE EXERCISES

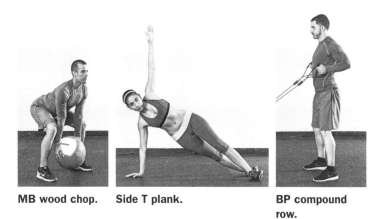

MB wood chop.   Side T plank.   BP compound row.

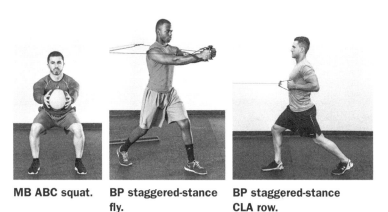

MB ABC squat.   BP staggered-stance fly.   BP staggered-stance CLA row.

THE HOW

If your fitness level is high, you can start with any week that feels comfortable and repeat the week as many times as necessary to create a strong base of training.

TABLE 9.4 Racket Sports: Conditioning Triplexes

Exercise	Week 1	Week 2	Week 3	Week 4	Page
Triplex 1 1. MB wood chop 2. Side T plank 3. BP compound row	2 × 10	3 × 10	3 × 15	4 × 10 to 15	110 58 80
Triplex 2 1. MB ABC squat 2. BP staggered-stance fly 3. BP staggered-stance CLA row	2 × 10	3 × 10	3 × 15	4 × 10 to 15	112 76 81

Core 1

Core Activator: 2 × 10

Rope circles (clockwise and counterclockwise): 2 × 10 to 15 sec. each direction

Vibration blade throw: 2 × 10 sec. per side

STRENGTH

Perform each triplex in order for the number of sets indicated. Rest adequately between each exercise to maintain good form and quality of movement, eventually targeting a 30- to 60-second rest period after each exercise. Use enough load to make the assigned repetitions challenging while maintaining good form. Unless otherwise specified, use the progression in table 9.5.

THE EXERCISES

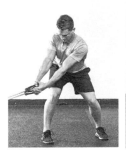
BP low-to-high chop.

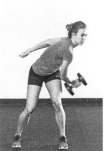
DB single-arm diagonal fly rotation.

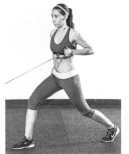
BP staggered-stance CLA compound row.

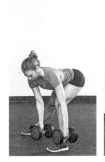
DB or KB lateral reaching lunge.

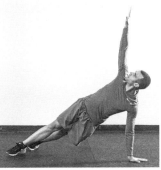
T push-up.

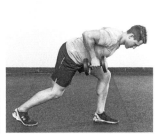
DB or KB staggered-stance bent-over single-arm row.

> continued

THE HOW

If your fitness level is high, you can start with any week that feels comfortable and repeat the week as many times as necessary to create a strong base of training.

TABLE 9.5 Racket Sports: Strength Triplexes

The DB single-arm diagonal fly rotation and DB or KB staggered-stance bent-over single-arm row should be performed on each arm.

Exercise	Week 1	Week 2	Week 3	Week 4	Page
Triplex 1	1 × 6	2 × 6	3 × 4	4 × 4	
1. BP low-to-high chop					86
2. DB single-arm diagonal fly rotation					106
3. BP staggered-stance CLA compound row					83
Triplex 2	1 × 6	2 × 6	3 × 4	4 × 4	
1. DB or KB lateral reaching lunge					95
2. T push-up (slow)					60
3. DB or KB staggered-stance bent-over single-arm row					97

Core 2

X-up: 2 × 10

SB rollout: 2 × 10

Rope circles (clockwise and counterclockwise): 2 × 20 sec. each direction

Vibration blade throw: 2 × 15 sec. per side

POWER AND POWER ENDURANCE

Perform each biplex in order for the number of sets indicated. For power, rest 1 minute between the first and second exercises and then 1 to 2 minutes between the second and first exercises. For power endurance, do not rest between the first and second exercises, but rest 1 minute between the second and first exercises. Use enough load to make the assigned repetitions challenging while maintaining good form. Unless otherwise specified, use the progression in table 9.6.

Additional Warm-Up

Crooked stick hexagon drill: 2 or 3 sets

Crooked stick cross-rotational jump drill: 2 or 3 sets

THE EXERCISES

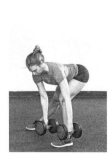

DB or KB lateral reaching lunge.

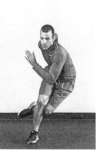

Skater.

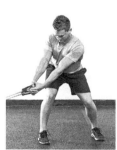

BP low-to-high chop.

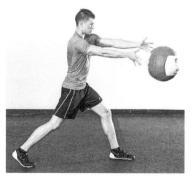

MB rotational throw: perpendicular.

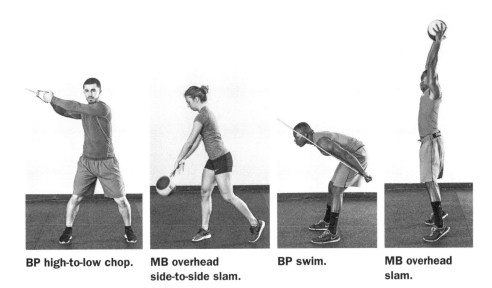

BP high-to-low chop.

MB overhead side-to-side slam.

BP swim.

MB overhead slam.

THE HOW

If your fitness level is high, you can start with any week that feels comfortable and repeat the week as many times as necessary to create a strong base of training.

TABLE 9.6 Racket Sports: Power and Power-Endurance Biplexes

Exercise	Week 1	Week 2	Week 3	Week 4	Page
Biplex 1 1. DB or KB lateral reaching lunge 2. Skater	2 × 5 + 5	3 × 5 + 5	3 or 4 × 5 + 5	4 × 5 + 5	95 67
Biplex 2 1. BP low-to-high chop 2. MB rotational throw: perpendicular	2 × 5 + 5	3 × 5 + 5	3 or 4 × 5 + 5	4 × 5 + 5	86 121
Biplex 3 1. BP high-to-low chop 2. MB overhead side-to-side slam	2 × 5 + 5	3 × 5 + 5	3 or 4 × 5 + 5	4 × 5 + 5	85 121
Biplex 4 1. BP swim 2. MB overhead slam	2 × 5 + 5	3 × 5 + 5	3 or 4 × 5 + 5	4 × 5 + 5	84 120

5 + 5 indicates 60 seconds of rest between the first and second exercise for power. For power endurance, go straight from the first exercise to the second without resting.

Core 3

Single-leg CLA anterior reach: 3 × 10 per leg

Rope circles (clockwise and counterclockwise): 3 × 10 to 15 sec. each direction

Vibration blade throw: 3 × 10 sec. per side

Metabolic

For power: spider drill, 2 or 3 sets, 3 times per week (1:3 work:rest ratio)

For power endurance: spider drill, 4 or 5 sets, 2 or 3 times per week (1:2 to 1:1 work:rest ratio)

Aim to complete the spider drill in 17 to 21 seconds.

Sports such as baseball, softball, and cricket consist primarily of batting, throwing, and catching. Batting requires strong rotational movements and force transfer from the ground to the arms. The throwing motion uses the anterior aspect of the core to generate power. Catching requires various abilities, depending on the sport and position the athlete plays. A power-endurance phase is included for high-repetition positions such as pitchers and catchers.

Warm-Up for Conditioning and Strength

Gary's Dumbbell Matrix: 1 or 2 sets

Vibration blade throw: 3 × 10 per side

CONDITIONING

Perform each triplex in order and then start the sequence again. Complete as many sets as indicated. Rest adequately between each exercise to maintain good form and quality of movement, eventually targeting a 30- to 60-second rest period after each exercise. Use enough load to make the assigned repetitions challenging while maintaining good form. Unless otherwise specified, use the progression in table 9.7.

THE EXERCISES

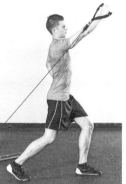

MB wood chop.

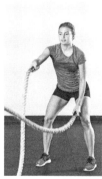

BP staggered-stance CLA incline press.

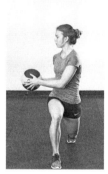

Ropes alternating up and down.

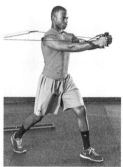

MB lunge with rotation.

BP staggered-stance fly.

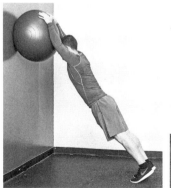

SB rollout.

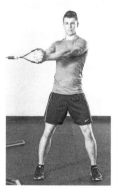

BP high-to-low chop.

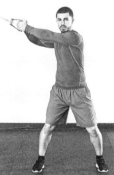

BP short rotation (10 to 2 o'clock).

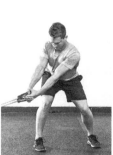

BP low-to-high chop.

THE HOW

If your fitness level is high, you can start with any week that feels comfortable and repeat the week as many times as necessary to create a strong base of training.

TABLE 9.7 Batting, Throwing, and Catching Sports: Conditioning Triplexes

Exercise	Week 1	Week 2	Week 3	Week 4	Page
Triplex 1 1. MB wood chop 2. BP staggered-stance CLA incline press 3. Ropes alternating up and down	2 × 10	3 × 10	3 × 15	4 × 10 to 15	110 73 139
Triplex 2 1. MB lunge with rotation 2. BP staggered-stance fly 3. SB rollout	2 × 10	3 × 10	3 × 15	4 × 10 to 15	113 76 127
Triplex 3 (Steel Core) 1. BP high-to-low chop 2. BP short rotation (10 to 2 o'clock) 3. BP low-to-high chop	2 × 10	3 × 10	3 × 15	4 × 10 to 15	85 87 86

Core 1

Fabulous Five: 2 sets

Vibration blade throw: 2 × 10 sec. per side

Rope circles (clockwise and counterclockwise): 2 × 10 sec. each direction

STRENGTH

Perform each triplex in order for the number of sets indicated. Rest adequately between each exercise to maintain good form and quality of movement, eventually targeting a 30- to 60-second rest period after each exercise. Use enough load to make the assigned repetitions challenging while maintaining good form. Unless otherwise specified, use the progression in table 9.8.

THE EXERCISES

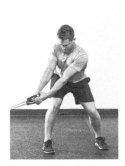
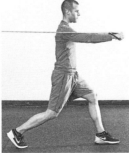
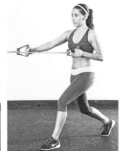

BP low-to-high chop.   **BP staggered-stance CLA press.**   **BP staggered-stance alternating row.**

> continued

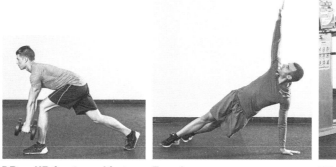

DB or KB front reaching lunge.

T push-up.

BP push–pull.

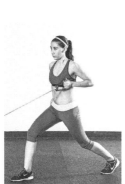
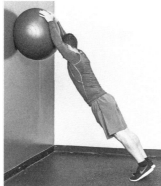
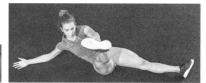

BP staggered-stance CLA compound row.

SB rollout.

X-up.

THE HOW

If your fitness level is high, you can start with any week that feels comfortable and repeat the week as many times as necessary to create a strong base of training.

TABLE 9.8 Batting, Throwing, and Catching Sports: Strength Triplexes

Exercise	Week 1	Week 2	Week 3	Week 4	Page
Triplex 1	1 × 6	2 × 6	3 × 4	4 × 4	
1. BP low-to-high chop					86
2. BP staggered-stance CLA press					72
3. BP staggered-stance alternating row					78
Triplex 2	1 × 6	2 × 6	3 × 4	4 × 4	
1. DB or KB front reaching lunge					94
2. T push-up (slow)					60
3. BP push–pull					89
Triplex 3	1 × 6	2 × 6	3 × 4	4 × 4	
1. BP staggered-stance CLA compound row					83
2. SB rollout					127
3. X-up*					62

*Make the exercise harder by slowing down to a 3 count up and 3 count down.

Core 2

Ropes alternating up and down: 2 × 20 per arm

Rope circles (clockwise and counterclockwise): 2 × 10 to 20 sec. each direction

Vibration blade throw: 2 × 10 sec. each side

POWER AND POWER ENDURANCE

Perform each biplex in order for the number of sets indicated. For power, rest 1 minute between the first and second exercises, and then rest 1 to 2 minutes between the second and first exercises. For power endurance, do not rest between the first and second exercises, and then rest 1 minute between the second and first exercises. Use enough load to make the assigned repetitions challenging while maintaining good form. Unless otherwise specified, use the progression shown in table 9.9.

Warm-Up

Steel Core: 3 × 10

Ropes alternating up and down: 2 × 20 per arm

Rope circles (clockwise and counterclockwise): 2 × 10 to 20 sec. each direction

THE EXERCISES

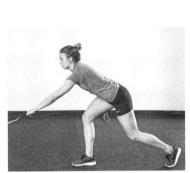

BP staggered-stance CLA deadlift.

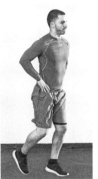

Alternating split jump.

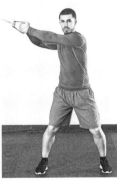

BP high-to-low chop.

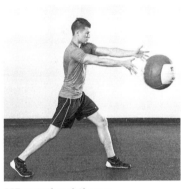

MB rotational throw: perpendicular.

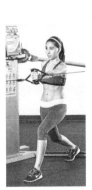

BP push–pull.

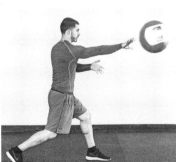

MB staggered-stance CLA straight chest throw.

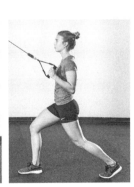

BP staggered-stance CLA high-to-low row.

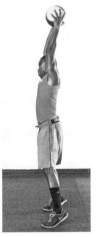

MB overhead slam.

> continued

THE HOW

If your fitness level is high, you can start with any week that feels comfortable and repeat the week as many times as necessary to create a strong base of training.

TABLE 9.9   Batting, Throwing, and Catching Sports: Power and Power-Endurance Biplexes

Exercise	Week 1	Week 2	Week 3	Week 4	Page
POWER					
Biplex 1 1. BP staggered-stance CLA deadlift 2. Alternating split jump	2 × 5 + 5	2 × 5 + 5	3 × 5 + 5	3 × 5 + 5	71 66
Biplex 2 1. BP high-to-low chop 2. MB rotational throw: perpendicular	2 × 5 + 5	2 × 5 + 5	3 × 5 + 5	3 × 5 + 5	85 121
Biplex 3 1. BP push–pull 2. MB staggered-stance CLA straight chest throw	2 × 5 + 5	2 × 5 + 5	3 × 5 + 5	3 × 5 + 5	89 118
Biplex 4 1. BP staggered-stance CLA high-to-low row 2. MB overhead slam	2 × 5 + 5	2 × 5 + 5	3 × 5 + 5	3 × 5 + 5	82 120
POWER ENDURANCE					
Biplex 1 1. BP staggered-stance CLA deadlift 2. Alternating split jump	2 or 3 × 5 + 5	2 or 3 × 5 + 5	3 or 4 × 5 + 5	3 or 4 × 5 + 5	71 66
Biplex 2 1. BP high-to-low chop 2. MB rotational throw: perpendicular	2 or 3 × 5 + 5	2 or 3 × 5 + 5	3 or 4 × 5 + 5	3 or 4 × 5 + 5	85 121
Biplex 3 1. BP push–pull 2. MB staggered-stance CLA straight chest throw	2 or 3 × 5 + 5	2 or 3 × 5 + 5	3 or 4 × 5 + 5	3 or 4 × 5 + 5	89 118
Biplex 4 1. BP staggered-stance CLA high-to-low row 2. MB overhead slam	2 or 3 × 5 + 5	2 or 3 × 5 + 5	3 or 4 × 5 + 5	3 or 4 × 5 + 5	82 120

5 + 5 indicates 60 seconds of rest between the first and second exercise for power. For power endurance, go straight from the first exercise to the second without resting.

Core 3

SB rollout: 3 × 10

Single-leg CLA anterior reach: 3 × 10 per leg

Vibration blade throw: 2 × 10 sec. each side

Sports that require high power or sustained running, such as track and field and endurance running, are rarely grouped together. However, all running is a variation of a sprint. This approach is substantiated by the increased amount of forefoot running in long races (e.g., mile, 5K, marathons). Long distances that used to be covered using a heel-to-toe (full foot) plant are now being raced on the forefoot and finished in sprint times. Therefore, this program increases the power output of the body's locomotive system and then lets the athlete adapt the power gained to his specific race and distance covered.

Warm-Up for Conditioning and Strength

Fabulous Five: 2 sets

Runner's reach: 2 × 10 to 20

Slide running: 2 × 10 per side

CONDITIONING

Perform each quadplex in order and then start the sequence again. Complete for as many sets as indicated. Rest adequately between each exercise to maintain good form and quality of movement, eventually targeting a 30- to 60-second rest period after each exercise. Use enough load to make the assigned repetitions challenging while maintaining good form. Unless otherwise specified, use the progression in table 9.10.

THE EXERCISES

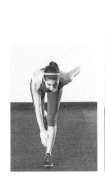
Single-leg CLA anterior reach.

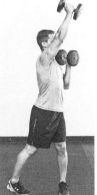
DB or KB cross overhead press.

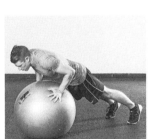
SB hands-on-ball push-up.

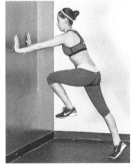
45-degree calf pump.

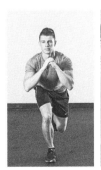
Single-leg squat.

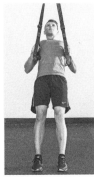
BP push–pull.

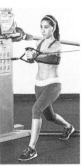
Recline pull (row).

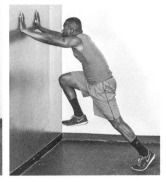
45-degree wall run.

> continued

THE HOW

If your fitness level is high, you can start with any week that feels comfortable and repeat the week as many times as necessary to create a strong base of training.

TABLE 9.10   Running Sports: Conditioning Quadplexes

The single-leg CLA anterior reach and single-leg squat should be performed on each leg.

Exercise	Week 1	Week 2	Week 3	Week 4	Page
Quadplex 1 1. Single-leg CLA anterior reach 2. DB or KB cross overhead press 3. SB hands-on-ball push-up 4. 45-degree calf pump (15 sec.)	2 × 10	3 × 10	3 × 15	4 × 10 to 15	39 100 125 63
Quadplex 2 1. Single-leg squat 2. BP push–pull 3. Recline pull (row) 4. 45-degree wall run (15 sec.)	2 × 10	3 × 10	3 × 15	4 × 10 to 15	40 89 46 64

Core 1

Triple Threat (weeks 1-5)

Running curl: 2 or 3 × 10 to 20 per arm

STRENGTH

Perform each triplex in order for the number of sets indicated. Rest adequately between each exercise to maintain good form and quality of movement, eventually targeting a 30- to 60-second rest period after each exercise. Use enough load to make the assigned repetitions challenging while keeping good form. Unless otherwise specified, use the progression in table 9.11.

Additional Warm-Up

45-degree calf pump: 2 × 30 sec.

45-degree wall run: 2 × 30 sec.

THE EXERCISES

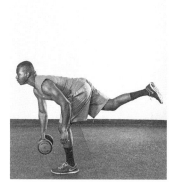

DB or KB single-leg RDL.

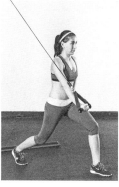

BP staggered-stance CLA decline press.

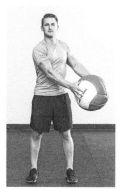

MB short diagonal chop.

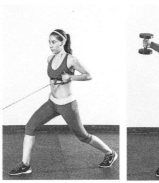

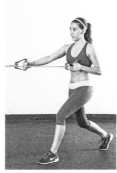

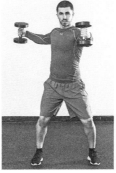

BP staggered-stance CLA compound row.

DB horizontal fly rotation.

BP staggered-stance alternating row.

THE HOW

If your fitness level is high, you can start with any week that feels comfortable and repeat the week as many times as necessary to create a strong base of training.

TABLE 9.11 Running Sports: Strength Triplexes

The DB or KB single-leg RDL should be performed on each leg.

Exercise	Week 1	Week 2	Week 3	Week 4	Page
Triplex 1 1. DB or KB single-leg RDL 2. BP staggered-stance CLA decline press 3. MB short diagonal chop	2 × 6	3 × 6	3 × 4	4 × 4	92 74 112
Triplex 2 1. BP staggered-stance CLA compound row 2. DB horizontal fly rotation 3. BP staggered-stance alternating row	2 × 6	3 × 6	3 × 4	4 × 4	83 105 78

Core 2

Triple Threat (weeks 6-10)

Running curl: 2 or 3 × 10 to 20 per arm

Ropes alternating up and down: 2 or 3 × 10 to 20 per arm

POWER AND POWER ENDURANCE

Perform each quadplex in order and then start the sequence again. Complete for as many sets as indicated. For power, rest 1 minute between exercises and then 1 to 2 minutes between the second and first exercises. For power endurance, do not rest between exercises and then rest 0 to 30 seconds between circuits. Use enough load to make the assigned repetitions challenging while maintaining good form. Unless otherwise specified, use the progression in table 9.12.

Warm-Up

45-degree calf pump: 2 or 3 × 45 to 60 sec.

45-degree wall run: 2 or 3 × 45 to 60 sec.

Runner's reach: 2 × 10 to 20

Slide running: 2 × 10 per side

> continued

THE EXERCISES

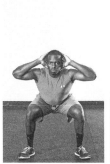
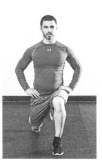
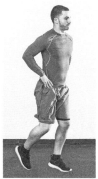
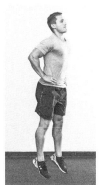

Bodyweight double-leg squat. **Bodyweight alternating lunge.** **Alternating split jump.** **Squat jump.**

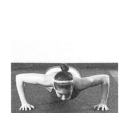
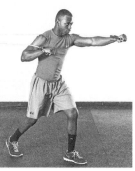
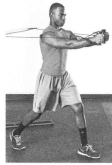
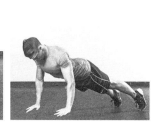

Bodyweight push-up. **BP staggered-stance alternating press.** **BP staggered-stance fly.** **Explosive push-up.**

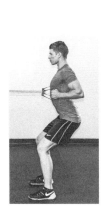
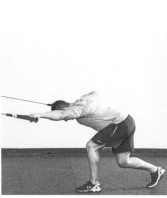
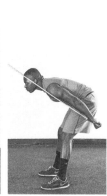
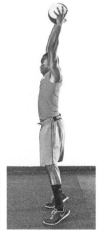

BP row. **BP staggered-stance bent-over alternating row.** **BP swim.** **MB overhead slam.**

THE HOW

If your fitness level is high, you can start with any week that feels comfortable and repeat the week as many times as necessary to create a strong base of training.

TABLE 9.12 Running Sports: Power and Power-Endurance Complexes

	POWER*				
Exercise	**Week 1**	**Week 2**	**Week 3**	**Week 4**	**Page**
Meta complex 1	2 sets	2 sets	3 sets	3 sets	
(JC Leg Crank)					
Bodyweight double-leg squat	× 24	× 24	× 24	× 24	42
Bodyweight alternating lunge	× 12 per leg	× 12 per leg	× 12 per leg	× 12 per leg	43
Alternating split jump	× 12 per leg	× 12 per leg	× 12 per leg	× 12 per leg	66
Squat jump	× 12	× 12	× 12	× 12	66
Meta complex 2	2 sets	2 sets	3 sets	3 sets	
(JC Meta Chest 1.0)					
Bodyweight push-up	× 20	× 20	× 20	× 20	44
BP staggered-stance alternating press	× 20 per leg	× 20 per leg	× 20 per leg	× 20 per leg	75
BP staggered-stance fly	× 10 per side	× 10 per side	× 10 per side	× 10 per side	76
Explosive push-up	× 10	× 10	× 10	× 10	69
Meta complex 3	2 sets	2 sets	3 sets	3 sets	
(JC Meta Back)					
BP row	× 20	× 20	× 20	× 20	77
BP staggered-stance bent-over alternating row	× 20 per arm and leg	× 20 per arm and leg	× 20 per arm and leg	× 20 per arm and leg	79
BP swim	× 20	× 20	× 20	× 20	84
MB overhead slam	× 10	× 10	× 10	× 10	120
	POWER ENDURANCE**				
Meta complex 1	2 sets	2 sets	3 sets	3 sets	
(JC Leg Crank)					
Bodyweight double-leg squat	× 24	× 24	× 24	× 24	42
Bodyweight alternating lunge	× 12 per leg	× 12 per leg	× 12 per leg	× 12 per leg	43
Alternating split jump	× 12 per leg	× 12 per leg	× 12 per leg	× 12 per leg	66
Squat jump	× 12	× 12	× 12	× 12	66
Meta complex 2	1 to 2 sets	1 to 2 sets	2 sets	2 sets	
(JC Meta Chest 1.0)					
Bodyweight push-up	× 20	× 20	× 20	× 20	44
BP staggered-stance alternating press	× 20 per leg	× 20 per leg	× 20 per leg	× 20 per leg	75
BP staggered-stance fly	× 10 per side	× 10 per side	× 10 per side	× 10 per side	76
Explosive push-up	× 10	× 10	× 10	× 10	69
Meta complex 3	1 to 2 sets	1 to 2 sets	3 sets	3 sets	
(JC Meta Back)					
BP row	× 20	× 20	× 20	× 20	77
BP staggered-stance bent-over alternating row	× 20 per arm and leg	× 20 per arm and leg	× 20 per arm and leg	× 20 per arm and leg	79
BP swim	× 20	× 20	× 20	× 20	84
MB overhead slam	× 10	× 10	× 10	× 10	120

*During the power phase, rest 30-60 seconds between each exercise and 1-2 minutes between each circuit. Concentrate on high intensity with each repetition.

**During the power endurance phase, do not rest between each exercise. During weeks 1 and 2, rest 1 minute between each circuit. During week 3, rest only 30 seconds between each circuit. Week 4, try not to rest between exercises or sets.

Supplemental Core

Triple Threat (weeks 11-15) for power
Triple Threat (weeks 16-20) for power endurance
Running curl: 2 or 3 × 10 to 20 per arm
Ropes alternating up and down: 2 or 3 × 10 to 20 per arm

Combat sports, such as mixed martial arts (MMA), judo, wrestling, and taekwondo, require a combination of power and endurance. The contractions needed for combat can range from long isometric contractions to short, explosive muscle actions. Regardless of grappling or striking technique, strong rotational forces traveling through the core are the key characteristic targeted for improvement.

Warm-Up for All Workouts

Gary's Dumbbell Matrix: 2 or 3 sets, dumbbells (5-10 percent of body weight)

CONDITIONING

Perform each quadplex in order and then start the sequence again. Complete for as many sets as indicated. Rest adequately between each exercise to maintain good form and quality of movement, eventually targeting a 30- to 60-second rest period after each exercise. Use enough load to make the assigned repetitions challenging while maintaining good form. Unless otherwise specified, use the progression in table 9.13.

THE EXERCISES

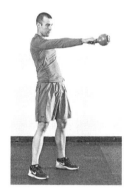
KB single-arm swing.

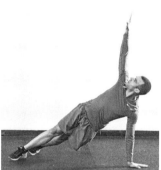
T push-up.

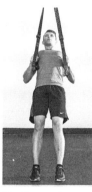
Recline pull (row).

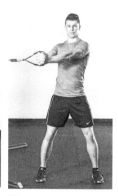
BP short rotation (10 to 2 o'clock).

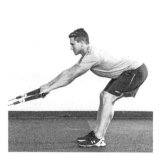
BP deadlift.

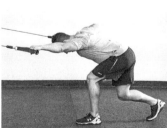
BP staggered-stance bent-over alternating row.

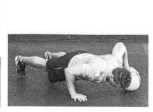
MB crossover push-up.

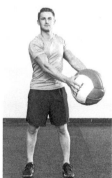
MB short diagonal chop.

THE HOW

If your fitness level is high, you can start with any week that feels comfortable and repeat the week as many times as necessary to create a strong base of training.

TABLE 9.13 Combat Sports: Conditioning Quadplexes

The KB single-arm swing should be performed on each arm.

Exercise	Week 1	Week 2	Week 3	Week 4	Page
Quadplex 1	2 × 10	3 × 10	3 × 15	4 × 10 to 15	
1. KB single-arm swing					91
2. T push-up					60
3. Recline pull (row)					46
4. BP short rotation (10 to 2 o'clock)					87
Quadplex 2	2 × 10	3 × 10	3 × 15	4 × 10 to 15	
1. BP deadlift					70
2. BP staggered-stance bent-over alternating row					79
3. MB crossover push-up					115
4. MB short diagonal chop					112

Core 1

DB or KB carry: 2 or 3 × 30 sec.

Ropes alternating up and down: 2 × 20 per arm

Rope circles (clockwise and counterclockwise): 2 × 10 to 20 sec. each direction

STRENGTH

Perform each quadplex in order and then start the sequence again. Rest adequately between each exercise to maintain good form and quality of movement, eventually targeting a 30- to 60-second rest period after each exercise. Use enough load to make the assigned repetitions challenging while maintaining good form. Unless otherwise specified, use the progression in table 9.14.

THE EXERCISES

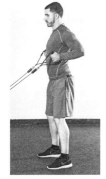

BP compound row.

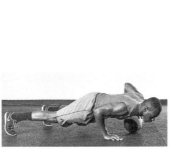

MB single-arm push-off.

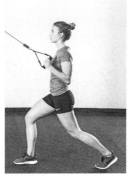

BP staggered-stance CLA high-to-low row.

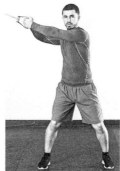

BP high-to-low chop.

> continued

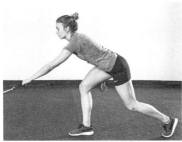

BP staggered-stance CLA deadlift.

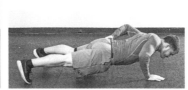

Single-arm eccentrics.

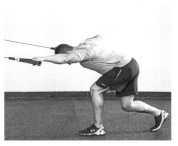

BP staggered-stance bent-over alternating row.

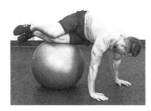

SB skier.

THE HOW

If your fitness level is high, you can start with any week that feels comfortable and repeat the week as many times as necessary to create a strong base of training.

TABLE 9.14 Combat Sports: Strength Quadplexes

The MB single-arm push-off and single-arm eccentrics should be performed on each arm.

Exercise	Week 1	Week 2	Week 3	Week 4	Page
Quadplex 1	1 × 6	2 × 6	3 × 4	4 × 4	
1. BP compound row					80
2. MB single-arm push-off					114
3. BP staggered-stance CLA high-to-low row					82
4. BP high-to-low chop					85
Quadplex 2	1 × 6	2 × 6	3 × 4	4 × 4	
1. BP staggered-stance CLA deadlift					71
2. Single-arm eccentrics					59
3. BP staggered-stance bent-over alternating row					79
4. SB skier					132

Core 2

DB or KB carry: 4 × 30 sec.

Ropes alternating up and down: 3 × 20 per arm

Rope circles (clockwise and counterclockwise): 3 × 10 to 20 sec. each direction

POWER

Perform each biplex in order and then start the sequence again. Rest for 1 minute between the first and second exercises and then 1 to 2 minutes between the second and first exercises. Use enough load to make the assigned repetitions challenging while maintaining good form. Unless otherwise specified, use the progression in table 9.15.

THE EXERCISES

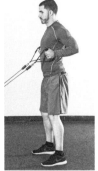

BP compound row.

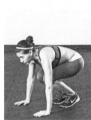

Burpee.

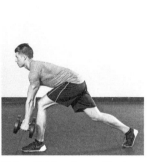

DB or KB front reaching lunge.

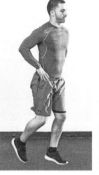

Alternating split jump.

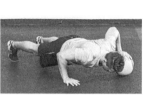

MB crossover push-up.

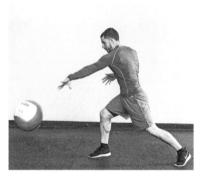

MB staggered-stance CLA decline chest throw.

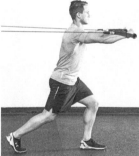

BP staggered-stance press.

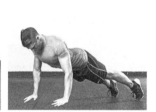

Explosive push-up.

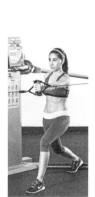

BP push–pull.

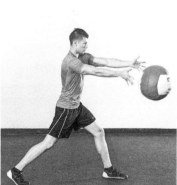

MB rotational throw.

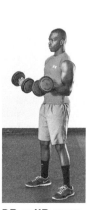

DB or KB carry.

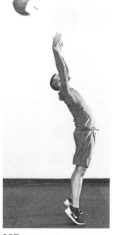

MB reverse scoop throw.

> *continued*

THE HOW

If your fitness level is high, you can start with any week that feels comfortable and repeat the week as many times as necessary to create a strong base of training.

TABLE 9.15   Combat Sports: Power Biplexes

Exercise	Week 1	Week 2	Week 3	Week 4	Page
Biplex 1 1. BP compound row 2. Burpee	2 × 5 + 5	2 × 5 + 5	3 × 5 + 5	3 × 5 + 5	 80 68
Biplex 2 1. DB or KB front reaching lunge 2. Alternating split jump	2 × 5 + 5	2 × 5 + 5	3 × 5 + 5	3 × 5 + 5	 94 66
Biplex 3 1. MB crossover push-up 2. MB staggered-stance CLA decline chest throw	2 × 5 + 5	2 × 5 + 5	3 × 5 + 5	3 × 5 + 5	 115 119
Biplex 4 1. BP staggered-stance press 2. Explosive push-up	2 × 5 + 5	2 × 5 + 5	3 × 5 + 5	3 × 5 + 5	 74 69
Biplex 5 1. BP push–pull 2. MB rotational throw	2 × 5 + 5	2 × 5 + 5	3 × 5 + 5	3 × 5 + 5	 89 121
Biplex 6 1. DB or KB carry 2. MB reverse scoop throw	2 × 5 + 5	2 × 5 + 5	3 × 5 + 5	3 × 5 + 5	 107 122

POWER ENDURANCE

If you're training three times per week, you can perform a combination of the power and power-endurance program, depending on the sport training volume. Here's an example:

Monday: power

Wednesday: power endurance

Friday: power or opposite sequence for the week

For the power-endurance program, perform all 12 exercises in a row as a single set. Do not rest between exercises. During week 1, rest 3 minutes between sets. During week 2, rest 2 minutes between sets. During weeks 3 and 4, rest 1 minute between sets. Use enough load to make the assigned repetitions challenging while maintaining good form. Unless otherwise specified, use the progression in table 9.16.

THE EXERCISES

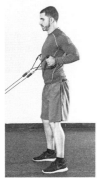

BP compound row.

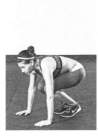

Burpee.

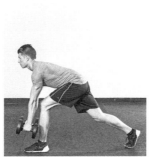

DB or KB front reaching lunge.

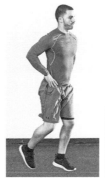

Alternating split jump.

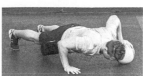

MB crossover push-up.

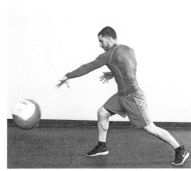

MB staggered-stance CLA decline chest throw.

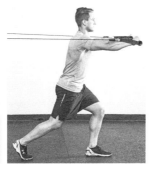

BP staggered-stance press.

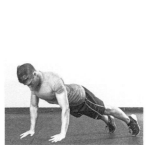

Explosive push-up.

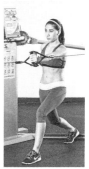

BP push–pull.

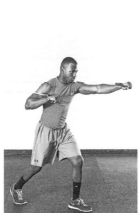

BP staggered-stance alternating press.

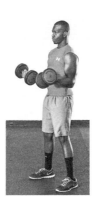

DB or KB carry.

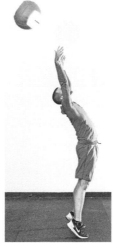

MB reverse scoop throw.

> continued

THE HOW

If your fitness level is high, you can start with any week that feels comfortable and repeat the week as many times as necessary to create a strong base of training. Try to complete as many repetitions as possible of each exercise in the time prescribed during the four-week progression, shooting for the following goals:

1. BP compound row: 25 reps in 25 seconds
2. Burpee: 10 to 15 reps in 25 seconds
3. DB or KB front reaching lunge: 8 to 12 reps per leg in 25 seconds
4. Alternating split jump: 12 reps per leg in 25 seconds
5. MB crossover push-up: 8 to 10 reps per side in 25 seconds
6. MB staggered-stance CLA decline chest throw: 6 to 9 reps per side in 25 seconds
7. BP staggered-stance press: 15 to 20 reps per leg in 25 seconds
8. Explosive push-up: 15 to 25 reps in 25 seconds
9. BP push–pull: 12 to 15 reps per side in 25 seconds
10. BP staggered-stance alternating press: 25 reps per leg in 25 seconds
11. DB or KB carry: 10 to 15 percent of body weight for 25 seconds
12. MB reverse scoop throw: 10 to 15 reps in 25 seconds

TABLE 9.16 Combat Sports: Power-Endurance Complex

Exercise	Week 1	Week 2	Week 3	Week 4	Page
Power-endurance superset	2 × 15 sec.	2 × 20 sec.	3 × 20 sec.	3 × 25 sec.	
1. BP compound row					80
2. Burpee					68
3. DB or KB front reaching lunge					94
4. Alternating split jump					66
5. MB crossover push-up					115
6. MB staggered-stance CLA decline chest throw					119
7. BP staggered-stance press					74
8. Explosive push-up					69
9. BP push–pull					89
10. BP staggered-stance alternating press					75
11. DB or KB carry					107
12. MB reverse scoop throw					122
Rest between sets	3 min.	2 min.	1 min.	1 min.	

Metabolic

Performing this circuit three to five times is enough metabolic training. If you need more, add two or three 300-yard (274 m) shuttles (25 yd [22.8 m] × 12) or other interval cardio training after you've completed all circuits. Practice and sparring volume must be taken into account when prescribing more metabolic training for combat athletes.

Long-distance field and court sports, such as soccer, lacrosse, handball, and kronum, use a combination of walking, jogging, explosive short sprints, jumping, and quick changes in direction. Total running distances can exceed 3 to 7 miles (5-11 km), depending on the sport and position. Although the total distance covered during a game is long, the short sprints rarely cover more than 15 to 20 yards (14-18 m) in a straight line. Body contact can range from light to intense, but it is sporadic and brief.

Warm-Up for All Workouts

Steel Core: 3 × 10

Single-leg CLA anterior reach: 3 × 10 to 20 per leg

Single-leg rotational squat: 3 × 10 per leg

CONDITIONING

Perform each triplex in order and then start the sequence again. Complete for as many sets as indicated. Rest adequately between each exercise to maintain good form and quality of movement, eventually targeting a 30- to 60-second rest period after each exercise. Use enough load to make the assigned repetitions challenging while maintaining good form. Unless otherwise specified, use the progression in table 9.17.

THE EXERCISES

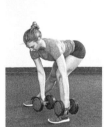

DB or KB lateral reaching lunge.

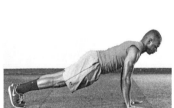

Plank.

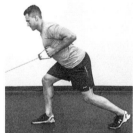

BP staggered-stance CLA low-to-high row.

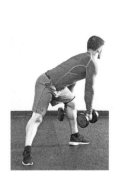

DB or KB rotating reaching lunge.

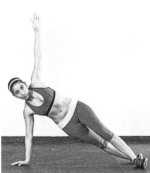

Side T plank.

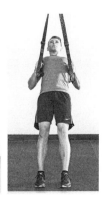

Recline pull (row).

> *continued*

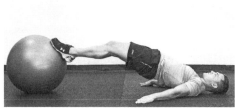
Triple Threat.

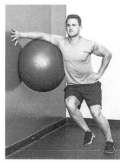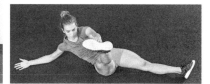
SB single-leg lateral wall slide. X-up.

THE HOW

If your fitness level is high, you can start with any week that feels comfortable and repeat the week as many times as necessary to create a strong base of training.

TABLE 9.17 Long-Distance Field and Court Sports: Conditioning Triplexes

Exercise	Week 1	Week 2	Week 3	Week 4	Page
Triplex 1					
1. DB or KB lateral reaching lunge	2 × 10	3 × 10	3 × 15	4 × 10 to 15	95
2. Plank (double-arm to single-arm progression)	10 to 30 sec.	10 to 30 sec.	10 to 30 sec.	10 to 30 sec.	57
3. BP staggered-stance CLA low-to-high row	2 × 10	3 × 10	3 × 15	4 × 10 to 15	82
Triplex 2					
1. DB or KB rotating reaching lunge	2 × 10	3 × 10	3 × 15	4 × 10 to 15	96
2. Side T plank	10 to 30 sec.	10 to 30 sec.	10 to 30 sec.	10 to 30 sec.	58
3. Recline pull (row)	2 × 10	3 × 10	3 × 15	4 × 10 to 15	46
Triplex 3 (core)					
1. Triple Threat (weeks 1-5)	2 × 10	3 × 10	3 × 15	4 × 10 to 15	185
2. SB single-leg lateral wall slide	3 × 10 per leg	3 × 10 per leg	3 × 10 per leg	3 × 10 per leg	124
3. X-up	3 × 10 per leg	3 × 10 per leg	3 × 10 per leg	3 ×σ 10 per leg	62

STRENGTH

Perform each triplex in order for the number of sets indicated. Rest adequately between each exercise to maintain good form and quality of movement, eventually targeting a 30- to 60-second rest period between each exercise. Use enough load to make the assigned repetitions challenging while maintaining good form. Unless otherwise specified, use the progression in table 9.18.

Additional Warm-Up

JC Leg Crank: 1 to 2 sets

Single-leg rotational squat: 2 ×s 10 per leg

THE EXERCISES

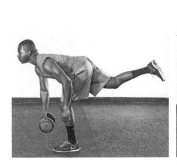

DB or KB single-leg RDL.

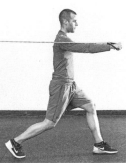

BP staggered-stance CLA press.

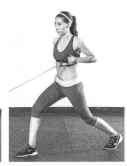

BP staggered-stance CLA compound row.

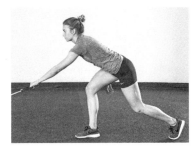

BP staggered-stance CLA deadlift.

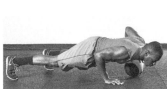

MB single-arm push-off.

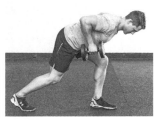

DB or KB staggered-stance bent-over single-arm row.

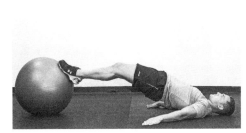

Triple Threat.

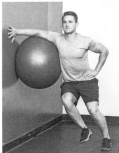

SB single-leg lateral wall slide.

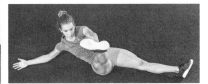

X-up.

THE HOW

If your fitness level is high, you can start with any week that feels comfortable and repeat the week as many times as necessary to create a strong base of training.

> continued

TABLE 9.18 Long-Distance Field and Court Sports: Strength Triplexes

The DB or KB single-leg RDL, MB single-arm push-off, and DB or KB staggered-stance bent-over single-arm row should be performed on each leg or arm.

Exercise	Week 1	Week 2	Week 3	Week 4	Page
Triplex 1 1. DB or KB single-leg RDL 2. BP staggered-stance CLA press 3. BP staggered-stance CLA compound row	2 × 6	2 × 6	3 to 4 × 4	3 to 4 × 4	92 72 83
Triplex 2 1. BP staggered-stance CLA deadlift 2. MB single-arm push-off 3. DB or KB staggered-stance bent-over single-arm row	2 × 6	2 × 6	3 to 4 × 4	3 to 4 × 4	71 114 97
Triplex 3 (core) 1. Triple Threat (weeks 1-5) 2. SB single-leg lateral wall slide 3. X-up	2 × 6 3 × 10 to 15 per leg 3 × 10 per leg	2 × 6 3 × 10 to 15 per leg 3 × 10 per leg	3 to 4 × 4 3 × 10 to 15 per leg 3 × 10 per leg	3 to 4 × 4 3 × 10 to 15 per leg 3 × 10 per leg	185 124 62

POWER

Perform each biplex in order for the number of sets indicated. Rest 1 minute between the first and second exercises, and then rest 1 to 2 minutes between the second and first exercises. Use enough load to make the assigned repetitions challenging while maintaining good form. Unless otherwise specified, use the progression in table 9.19.

Additional Warm-Up

JC Leg Crank: 1 or 2 sets

Low-hurdle run: 8 to 10 hurdles for 3 or 4 sets

Low-hurdle diagonal jump: 6 to 8 hurdles for 3 or 4 sets

THE EXERCISES

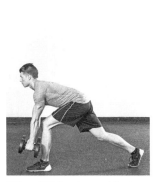

DB or KB front reaching lunge.

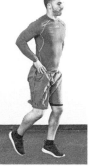

Alternating split jump.

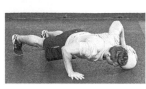

MB crossover push-up.

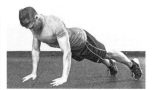

Explosive push-up.

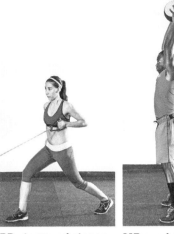
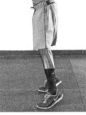
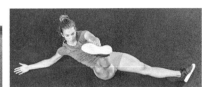
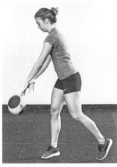

BP staggered-stance CLA compound row.

MB overhead slam.

X-up.

MB overhead side-to-side slam.

THE HOW

If your fitness level is high, you can start with any week that feels comfortable and repeat the week as many times as necessary to create a strong base of training.

TABLE 9.19 Long-Distance Field and Court Sports: Power Biplexes

Exercise	Week 1	Week 2	Week 3	Week 4	Page
Biplex 1 1. DB or KB front reaching lunge 2. Alternating split jump	2 or 3 × 5 + 5	2 or 3 × 5 + 5	3 or 4 × 5 + 5	3 or 4 × 5 + 5	94 66
Biplex 2 1. MB crossover push-up 2. Explosive push-up	2 or 3 × 5 + 5	2 or 3 × 5 + 5	3 or 4 × 5 + 5	3 or 4 × 5 + 5	115 69
Biplex 3 1. BP staggered-stance CLA compound row 2. MB overhead slam	2 or 3 × 5 + 5	2 or 3 × 5 + 5	3 or 4 × 5 + 5	3 or 4 × 5 + 5	83 120
Biplex 4 1. X-up 2. MB overhead side-to-side slam	2 or 3 × 5 + 5	2 or 3 × 5 + 5	3 or 4 × 5 + 5	3 or 4 × 5 + 5	62 121

Metabolic

300-yard (274 m) shuttle (25 yd [22.8 m] × 12): 2 or 3 sets 3 times per week (1:2 to 1:3 work:rest ratio)

Core

Triple Threat (weeks 11-15)

Single-leg CLA anterior reach: 2 × 10 to 20 per side

Single-leg rotational squat: 2 × 10 per side

> continued

POWER ENDURANCE

Perform each biplex in order for the number of sets indicated. Do not rest between the first and second exercises, and then rest 1 minute between the second and first exercises. Use enough load to make the assigned repetitions challenging while maintaining good form. Use specified repetitions and follow the progression in table 9.20.

Additional Warm-Up

Low-hurdle diagonal jump: 3 to 4 sets

Low-hurdle run: 3 to 4 sets

THE EXERCISES

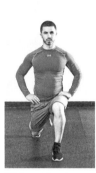

JC Leg Crank.

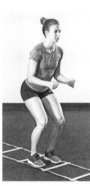

Agility ladder split step.

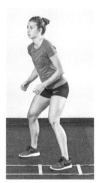

Agility ladder lateral rotational jump.

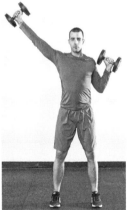

Gary's Dumbbell Matrix.

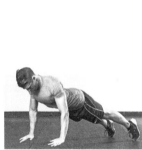

JC Meta Chest.

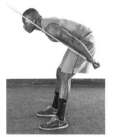

JC Meta Back.

THE HOW

If your fitness level is high, you can start with any week that feels comfortable and repeat the week as many times as necessary to create a strong base of training. On day 1, follow the power biplexes in table 9.19. On day 2, perform the power-endurance complexes in table 9.20.

TABLE 9.20 Long-Distance Field and Court Sports: Power-Endurance Complexes (Day 2)

Exercise	Week 1	Week 2	Week 3	Week 4	Page
Meta complex 1 JC Leg Crank Agility ladder split step (10 sec.) to agility ladder lateral rotational jump (10 sec.)	2 sets	2 sets	3 sets	3 sets	 187 134 135
Meta complex 2 Gary's Dumbbell Matrix: dumbbells 7 to 10 percent body weight; aim to complete all sets under 1:45 min	2 sets	2 sets	3 sets	3 sets	 190
Meta complex 3 JC Meta Chest	2 sets	2 sets	3 sets	3 sets	 189
Meta complex 4 JC Meta Back	2 sets	2 sets	3 sets	3 sets	 188
Work:rest ratio	1:2 to 1:3	1:2 to 1:3	1:1 to 1:2	1:1 to 1:2	

Metabolic

300-yard (274 m) shuttle (25 yd [22.8 m] × 12): 3 or 4 sets two times per week (1:2 to 1:1 work:rest ratio)

Core

Triple Threat (weeks 16-20)

Single-leg CLA anterior reach: 2 × 10 to 20 per side

Single-leg rotational squat: 2 × 10 per side

Volleyball is similar to sports such as racquetball in terms of low positions and baseball in terms of throwing. Players use a low position for digs and the throwing motion for serves or smashes. Many digs and saves end with a scramble from the ground, similar to movements found in wrestling and soccer. Quick and short changes of directions, especially lateral changes of direction, are needed during 5 to 8 seconds of all-out sprints, followed by 20 to 30 seconds of light to moderate intensity. The posterior musculature is particularly important due to these low positions and changes of directions.

Warm-Up for All Workouts

Gary's Dumbbell Matrix: 2 sets

CONDITIONING

Perform each triplex in order and then start the sequence again. Complete as many sets as indicated. Rest adequately between each exercise to maintain good form and quality of movement, eventually targeting a 30- to 60-second rest period between each exercise. Use enough load to make the assigned repetitions challenging while maintaining good form. Unless otherwise specified, use the progression in table 9.21.

THE EXERCISES

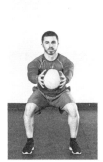

MB ABC squat.

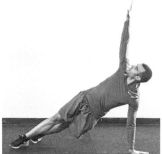

T push-up.

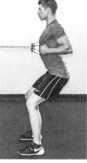

BP row.

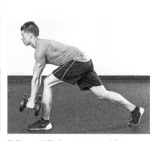

DB or KB front reaching lunge.

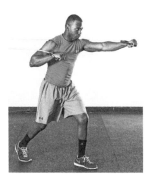

BP staggered-stance alternating press.

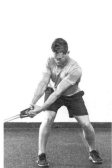

Recline pull (row).

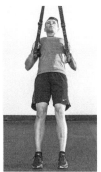

BP low-to-high chop.

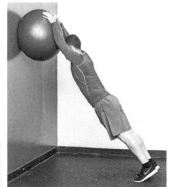

SB rollout.

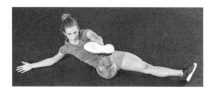

X-up.

THE HOW

If your fitness level is high, you can start with any week that feels comfortable and repeat the week as many times as necessary to create a strong base of training.

TABLE 9.21 Volleyball: Conditioning Triplexes

Exercise	Week 1	Week 2	Week 3	Week 4	Page
Triplex 1	2 × 10	3 × 10	3 × 15	4 × 10 to 15	
1. MB ABC squat					112
2. T push-up					60
3. BP row					77
Triplex 2	2 × 10	3 ×10	3 × 15	4 × 10 to 15	
1. DB or KB front reaching lunge					94
2. BP staggered-stance alternating press					75
3. Recline pull (row)					46
Triplex 3	2 × 10	3 × 10	3 × 15	4 × 10 to 15	
1. BP low-to-high chop					86
2. SB rollout					127
3. X-up					62

STRENGTH

Perform each triplex in order for the number of sets indicated. Rest adequately between each exercise to maintain good form and quality of movement, eventually targeting a 30- to 60-second rest period after each exercise. Use enough load to make the assigned repetition challenging while keeping good form. Unless otherwise specified, use the progression in table 9.22.

Warm-Up

Gary's Dumbbell Matrix: 1 set

SB rollout: 2 × 10

X-up: 2 × 10 per side

THE EXERCISES

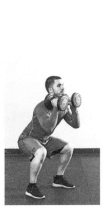
DB or KB squat.

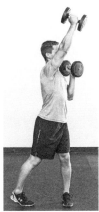
DB or KB cross overhead press.

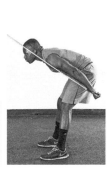
BP swim.

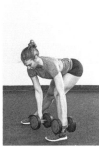
DB or KB lateral reaching lunge.

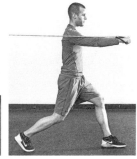
BP staggered-stance CLA press.

> continued

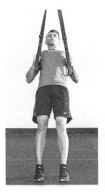

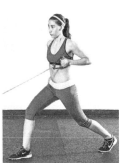

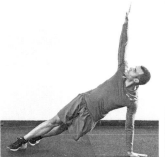

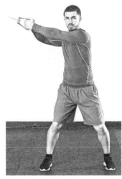

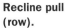

Recline pull (row).

BP staggered-stance CLA compound row.

T push-up.

BP high-to-low chop.

THE HOW

If your fitness level is high, you can start with any week that feels comfortable and repeat the week as many times as necessary to create a strong base of training.

TABLE 9.22 Volleyball: Strength Triplexes

Exercise	Week 1	Week 2	Week 3	Week 4	Page
Triplex 1	2 × 6	2 × 6	3 × 6	3 × 6	
1. DB or KB squat					90
2. DB or KB cross overhead press					100
3. BP swim					84
Triplex 2	2 × 6	2 × 6	3 × 6	3 × 6	
1. DB or KB lateral reaching lunge					95
2. BP staggered-stance CLA press					72
3. Recline pull (row)					46
Triplex 3	2 × 6	2 × 6	3 × 6	3 × 6	
1. BP staggered-stance CLA compound row					83
2. T push-up					60
3. BP high-to-low chop					85

POWER AND POWER ENDURANCE

Perform each biplex in order for the number of sets indicated. For power, rest 1 minute between the first and second exercises and then 1 to 2 minutes between the second and first exercises. For power endurance, do not rest between the first and second exercises, and then rest 1 minute between the second and first exercises. Use enough load to make the assigned repetitions challenging while maintaining good form. Unless otherwise specified, use the progression in table 9.23.

Warm-Up

Gary's Dumbbell Matrix: 1 set

SB rollout: 2 × 10

X-up: 2 × 10 per side

THE EXERCISES

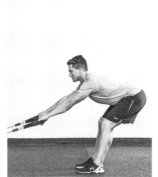

BP deadlift.

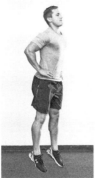

Vertical jump.

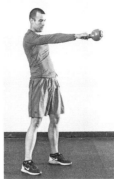

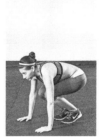

KB single-arm swing.

Burpee.

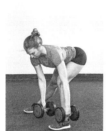

DB or KB lateral reaching lunge.

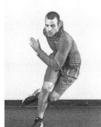

Skater.

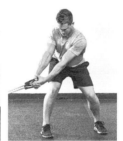

BP low-to-high chop.

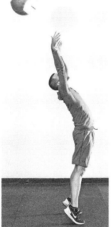

MB reverse scoop throw.

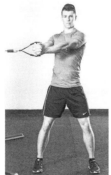

BP short rotation (10 to 2 o'clock).

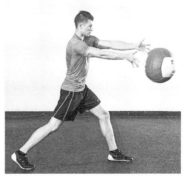

MB rotational throw: perpendicular.

> continued

THE HOW

If your fitness level is high, you can start with any week that feels comfortable and repeat the week as many times as necessary to create a strong base of training.

TABLE 9.23 Volleyball: Power and Power-Endurance Biplexes

The KB single-arm swing should be performed on each arm.

Exercise	Week 1	Week 2	Week 3	Week 4	Page
Biplex 1 1. BP deadlift 2. Vertical jump	2 × 5 + 5	2 × 5 + 5	3 × 5 + 5	3 × 5 + 5	70 65
Biplex 2 1. KB single-arm swing 2. Burpee	2 × 5 + 5	2 × 5 + 5	3 × 5 + 5	3 × 5 + 5	91 68
Biplex 3 1. DB or KB lateral reaching lunge 2. Skater	2 × 5 + 5	2 × 5 + 5	3 × 5 + 5	3 × 5 + 5	95 67
Biplex 4 1. BP low-to-high chop 2. MB reverse scoop throw	2 × 5 + 5	2 × 5 + 5	3 × 5 + 5	3 × 5 + 5	86 122
Biplex 5 1. BP short rotation (10 to 2 o'clock) 2. MB rotational throw: perpendicular	2 × 5 + 5	2 × 5 + 5	3 × 5 + 5	3 × 5 + 5	87 121

5 + 5 indicates 60 seconds of rest between the first and second exercise for power. For power endurance, go straight from the first exercise to the second without resting.

Metabolic

If you need more cardio or metabolic training during the power-endurance phase, add interval cardio, such as 300-yard (274 m) shuttles (25 yd [22.8 m] × 12), to the end of the workout. Practice volume must be taken into account when prescribing more metabolic training.

Golf is one of the most popular recreational sports in the world. It requires a high level of skill, pinpoint accuracy, rotational stability and power, and endurance during long playing time. Although power endurance is not often seen as a key attribute, we offered a power endurance program due to the fatigue that can be brought on by long playing times, often in hot climates. Many of the core stiffness and rotational qualities of baseball can be valuable in golf. Two-leg stability and hip rotation are essential.

Warm-Up for Conditioning and Strength

Gary's Dumbbell Matrix: 1 or 2 sets

BP pulsating backswing: 2 × 10 per side

BP high-to-low chop: 2 × 10 per side

BP short rotation (10 to 2 o'clock): 2 × 10 per side

CONDITIONING

Perform each triplex in order, and then start the sequence again. Complete as many sets as indicated. Rest adequately between each exercise to maintain good form and quality of movement, eventually targeting a 30-to 60-second rest period after each exercise. Use enough load to make the assigned repetitions challenging while maintaining good form. Unless otherwise specified, use the progression in table 9.24.

THE EXERCISES

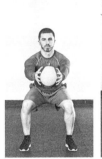

MB ABC squat.

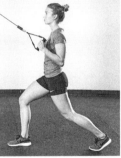

BP staggered-stance CLA high-to-low row.

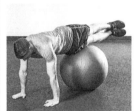

SB log roll.

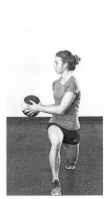

MB lunge with rotation.

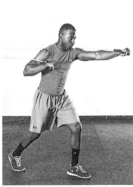

BP staggered-stance alternating press.

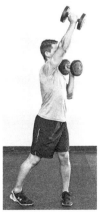

DB or KB cross overhead press.

> *continued*

THE HOW

If your fitness level is high, you can start with any week that feels comfortable and repeat the week as many times as necessary to create a strong base of training.

TABLE 9.24   Golf: Conditioning Triplexes

Exercise	Week 1	Week 2	Week 3	Week 4	Page
Triplex 1	2 × 10	3 × 10	3 × 15	4 × 10 to 15	
1. MB ABC squat					112
2. BP staggered-stance CLA high-to-low row					82
3. SB log roll					131
Triplex 2	2 × 10	3 × 10	3 × 15	4 × 10 to 15	
1. MB lunge with rotation					113
2. BP staggered-stance alternating press					75
3. DB or KB cross overhead press					100

Core 1

Fabulous Five: 2 sets

STRENGTH

Perform each triplex in order for the number of sets indicated. Rest adequately between each exercise to maintain good form and quality of movement, eventually targeting a 30- to 60-second rest period after each exercise. Use enough load to make the assigned repetitions challenging while maintaining good form. Unless otherwise specified, use the progression in table 9.25.

THE EXERCISES

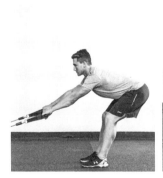

BP deadlift.

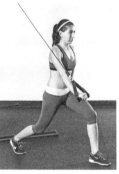

BP staggered-stance CLA decline press.

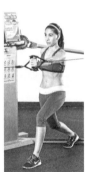

BP push–pull.

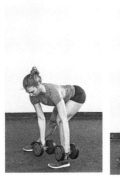
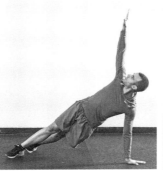
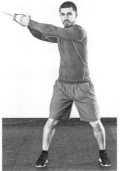

DB or KB lateral reaching lunge.   T push-up.   BP high-to-low chop.

THE HOW

If your fitness level is high, you can start with any week that feels comfortable and repeat the week as many times as necessary to create a strong base of training.

TABLE 9.25   Golf: Strength Triplexes

Exercise	Week 1	Week 2	Week 3	Week 4	Page
Triplex 1	1 × 6	2 × 6	3 × 4	4 × 4	
1. BP deadlift					70
2. BP staggered-stance CLA decline press					74
3. BP push–pull					89
Triplex 2	1 × 6	2 × 6	3 × 4	4 × 4	
1. DB or KB lateral reaching lunge					95
2. T push-up					60
3. BP high-to-low chop					85

Core 2

Fabulous Five: 2 sets

POWER AND POWER ENDURANCE

Perform each biplex in order for the number of sets indicated. For power, rest 1 minute between the first and second exercises, and then rest 1 to 2 minutes between the second and first exercises. For power endurance, do not rest between the first and second exercises, and then rest 1 minute between the second and first exercises. Use enough load to make the assigned repetitions challenging while maintaining good form. Unless otherwise specified, use the progression in table 9.26.

Warm-Up

Chopper: 2 sets

Gary's Dumbbell Matrix: 2 sets

> continued

THE EXERCISES

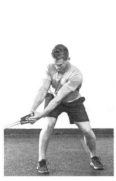

BP low-to-high chop.

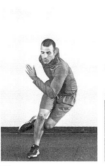

Skater.

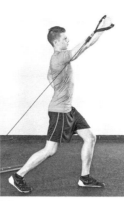

BP staggered-stance CLA incline press.

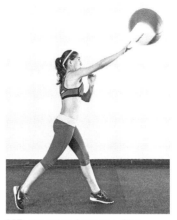

MB staggered-stance CLA incline chest throw.

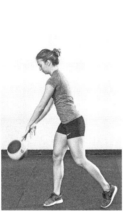

MB overhead side-to-side slam.

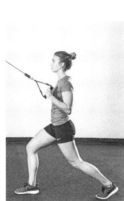

BP staggered-stance CLA high-to-low row.

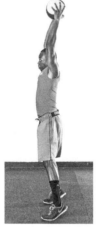

MB overhead slam.

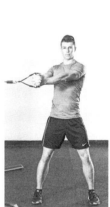

BP short rotation (10 to 2 o'clock).

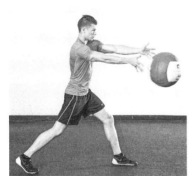

MB rotational throw: perpendicular.

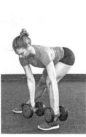

DB or KB lateral reaching lunge.

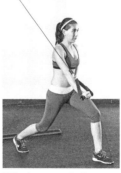

BP staggered-stance CLA decline press.

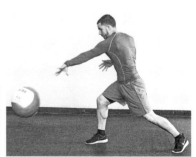

MB staggered-stance CLA decline chest throw.

THE HOW

If your fitness level is high, you can start with any week that feels comfortable and repeat the week as many times as necessary to create a strong base of training.

TABLE 9.26 Golf: Power and Power-Endurance Biplexes

POWER

Exercise	Week 1	Week 2	Week 3	Week 4	Page
Biplex 1 1. BP low-to-high chop 2. Skater	2 × 5 + 5	2 × 5 + 5	3 × 5 + 5	3 × 5 + 5	86 67
Biplex 2 1. BP staggered-stance CLA incline press 2. MB staggered-stance CLA incline chest throw	2 × 5 + 5	2 × 5 + 5	3 × 5 + 5	3 × 5 + 5	73 117
Biplex 3 1. BP staggered-stance CLA high-to-low row 2. MB overhead slam	2 × 5 + 5	2 × 5 + 5	3 × 5 + 5	3 × 5 + 5	82 120
Biplex 4 1. BP short rotation (10 to 2 o'clock) 2. MB rotational throw: perpendicular	2 × 5 + 5	2 × 5 + 5	3 × 5 + 5	3 × 5 + 5	87 121

POWER ENDURANCE

Exercise	Week 1	Week 2	Week 3	Week 4	Page
Biplex 1 1. DB or KB lateral reaching lunge 2. Skater	2 or 3 × 5 + 5	2 or 3 × 5 + 5	3 or 4 × 5 + 5	3 or 4 × 5 + 5	95 67
Biplex 2 1. BP staggered-stance CLA decline press 2. MB staggered-stance CLA decline chest throw	2 or 3 × 5 + 5	2 or 3 × 5 + 5	3 or 4 × 5 + 5	3 or 4 × 5 + 5	74 119
Biplex 3 1. BP staggered-stance CLA high-to-low row 2. MB overhead side-to-side slam	2 or 3 × 5 + 5	2 or 3 × 5 + 5	3 or 4 × 5 + 5	3 or 4 × 5 + 5	82 121
Biplex 4 1. BP short rotation (10 to 2 o'clock) 2. MB rotational throw: perpendicular	2 or 3 × 5 + 5	2 or 3 × 5 + 5	3 or 4 × 5 + 5	3 or 4 × 5 + 5	87 121

5 + 5 indicates 60 seconds of rest between the first and second exercise for power. For power endurance, go straight from the first exercise to the second without resting.

Core

BP pulsating backswing: 2 × 10 per side
SB log roll: 2 × 10 per side
Vibration blade 12 o'clock oscillation: 2 × 20 sec.

Board sports such as surfing and skateboarding are unique in that they use reaction forces between the athlete and the mass of the water or earth. Upper-body movements allow the lower body to manipulate the position of the board and the surface it interacts with. Strong legs and core muscles are needed to interact with the board and connect the lower body to the upper body. The upper body steers movement by changing lever arms and rotating the shoulders, directing forces down and onto the board. The bridge to all of this upper- and lower-body movement is the core.

Warm-Up for All Workouts

Chopper: 1 or 2 sets

Gary's Dumbbell Matrix: 1 or 2 sets

CONDITIONING

Perform each triplex in order, and then start the sequence again. Complete for as many sets as indicated. Rest adequately between each exercise to maintain good form and quality of movement, eventually targeting a 30- to 60-second rest period after each exercise. Use enough load to make the assigned repetitions challenging while maintaining good form. Unless otherwise specified, use the progression in table 9.27.

THE EXERCISES

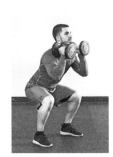

DB or KB squat.

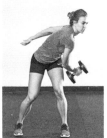

DB single-arm diagonal fly rotation.

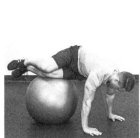

SB skier.

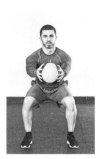

MB ABC squat.

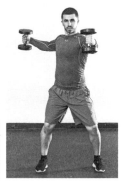

DB horizontal fly rotation.

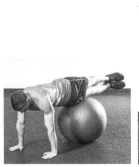

SB log roll.

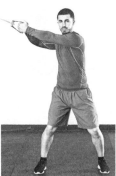

BP high-to-low chop.

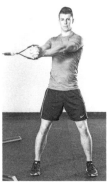

BP short rotation (10 to 2 o'clock).

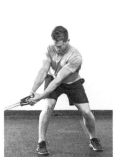

BP low-to-high chop.

THE HOW

If your fitness level is high, you can start with any week that feels comfortable and repeat the week as many times as necessary to create a strong base of training.

TABLE 9.27 Board Sports: Conditioning Triplexes

DB single-arm diagonal fly rotation should be performed on each arm.

Exercise	Week 1	Week 2	Week 3	Week 4	Page
Triplex 1 1. DB or KB squat 2. DB single-arm diagonal fly rotation 3. SB skier	2 × 10	2 × 15	3 × 15	4 × 10 to 15	90 106 132
Triplex 2 1. MB ABC squat 2. DB horizontal fly rotation 3. SB log roll	2 × 10	2 × 15	3 × 15	4 × 10 to 15	112 105 131
Triplex 3 (Steel Core) 1. BP high-to-low chop 2. BP short rotation (10 to 2 o'clock) 3. BP low-to-high chop	2 × 10	2 × 15	3 × 15	4 × 10 to 15	85 87 86

Core

Fabulous Five: 2 sets

STRENGTH

Perform each triplex in order for the number of sets indicated. Rest adequately between each exercise to maintain good form and quality of movement, eventually targeting a 30- to 60-second rest period after each exercise. Use enough load to make the assigned repetitions challenging while maintaining good form. Unless otherwise specified, use the progression in table 9.28.

THE EXERCISES

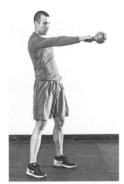 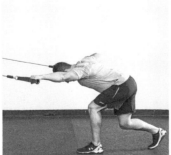 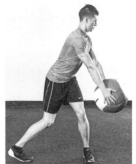

KB single-arm swing. **BP staggered-stance bent-over alternating row.** **MB diagonal chop.**

> continued

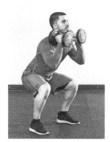

DB or KB squat.

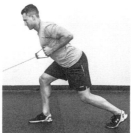

BP staggered-stance
CLA low-to-high row.

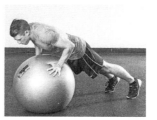

SB hands-on-ball push-up.

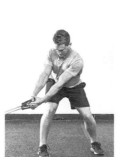

BP low-to-high chop.

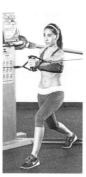

BP push–pull.

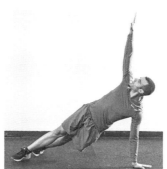

T push-up.

THE HOW

If your fitness level is high, you can start with any week that feels comfortable and repeat the week as many times as necessary to create a strong base of training.

TABLE 9.28 Board Sports: Strength Triplexes

The KB single-arm swing should be performed on each arm.

Exercise	Week 1	Week 2	Week 3	Week 4	Page
Triplex 1	2 × 6	2 × 6	3 × 4 to 6	3 × 4 to 6	
1. KB single-arm swing					91
2. BP staggered-stance bent-over alternating row					79
3. MB diagonal chop					111
Triplex 2	2 × 6	2 × 6	3 × 4 to 6	3 × 4 to 6	
1. DB or KB squat					90
2. BP staggered-stance CLA low-to-high row					82
3. SB hands-on-ball push-up (slow)					125
Triplex 3 (core)	2 × 6	2 × 6	3 × 4 to 6	3 × 4 to 6	
1. BP low-to-high chop					86
2. BP push–pull					89
3. T push-up (slow)					60

POWER AND POWER ENDURANCE

Perform each biplex in order for the number of sets indicated. For power, rest 1 minute between the first and second exercises, and then rest 1 to 2 minutes between the second and third exercises. For power endurance, do not rest between the first and second exercises, and then rest 1 minute between the second and first exercises. Use enough load to make the assigned repetitions challenging while maintaining good form. Unless otherwise specified, use the progression shown in table 9.29.

Additional Warm-Up

Steel Core: 2 or 3 × 10 to 15

THE EXERCISES

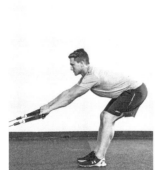

BP deadlift.

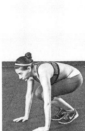

Burpee.

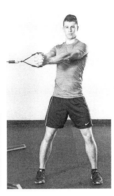

BP short rotation (10 to 2 o'clock).

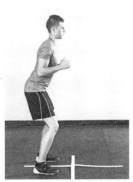

Crooked stick cross-rotational jump drill.

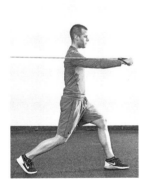

BP staggered-stance CLA press.

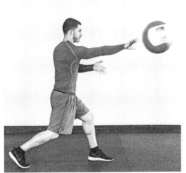

MB staggered-stance CLA straight chest throw.

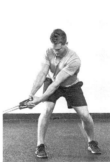

BP low-to-high chop.

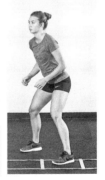

Agility ladder lateral rotational jump.

THE HOW

If your fitness level is high, you can start with any week that feels comfortable and repeat the week as many times as necessary to create a strong base of training.

> *continued*

TABLE 9.29   Board Sports: Power and Power-Endurance Biplexes

POWER					
Exercise	Week 1	Week 2	Week 3	Week 4	Page
Biplex 1 1. BP deadlift 2. Burpee	2 × 5 + 5	2 × 5 + 5	3 × 5 + 5	3 × 5 + 5	70 68
Biplex 2 1. BP short rotation (10 to 2 o'clock) 2. Crooked stick cross-rotational jump drill	2 × 5 + 5	2 × 5 + 5	3 × 5 + 5	3 × 5 + 5	87 138
Biplex 3 1. BP staggered-stance CLA press 2. MB staggered-stance CLA straight chest throw	2 × 5 + 5	2 × 5 + 5	3 × 5 + 5	3 × 5 + 5	72 118
Biplex 4 1. BP low-to-high chop 2. Agility ladder lateral rotational jump	2 × 5 + 5	2 × 5 + 5	3 × 5 + 5	3 × 5 + 5	86 135
POWER ENDURANCE					
Biplex 1 1. BP deadlift 2. Burpee	2 or 3 × 5 + 5	2 or 3 × 5 + 5	3 or 4 × 5 + 5	3 or 4 × 5 + 5	70 68
Biplex 2 1. BP short rotation (10 to 2 o'clock) 2. Crooked stick cross-rotational jump drill	2 or 3 × 5 + 5	2 or 3 × 5 + 5	3 or 4 × 5 + 5	3 or 4 × 5 + 5	87 138
Biplex 3 1. BP staggered-stance CLA press 2. MB staggered-stance CLA straight chest throw	2 or 3 × 5 + 5	2 or 3 × 5 + 5	3 or 4 × 5 + 5	3 or 4 × 5 + 5	72 118
Biplex 4 1. BP low-to-high chop 2. Agility ladder lateral rotational jump	2 or 3 × 5 + 5	2 or 3 × 5 + 5	3 or 4 × 5 + 5	3 or 4 × 5 + 5	86 135

5 + 5 indicates 60 seconds of rest between the first and second exercise for power. For power endurance, go straight from the first exercise to the second without resting.

Core

Fabulous Five: 2 sets

Metabolic

If you need more cardio or metabolic training in the power-endurance phase, add interval cardio, such as 300-yard (274 m) shuttles (25 yd [22.8 m] × 12), to the end of the workout. Practice volume must be taken into account when prescribing more metabolic training.

Power phase: JC Leg Crank, 2 sets with a 1:2 work:rest ratio

Power-endurance phase: JC Leg Crank, 3 or 4 sets with a 1:1 work:rest ratio

Swimming requires constant upper-body pulling power while maintaining a streamlined horizontal line. It's unique in that it does not involve ground reaction forces while in the water. The arms and legs are the main propulsion systems, and both are connected to and pull on the spine. This means the core is the anchor of all movement, and the back and legs can generate only the power that the core can support. For this reason, the core receives much attention in the swimming program.

Warm-Up for Conditioning and Strength

Chopper: 2 or 3 sets

CONDITIONING

Perform each quadplex in order, and then start the sequence again. Complete as many sets as indicated. Rest adequately between each exercise to maintain good form and quality of movement, eventually targeting a 30- to 60-second rest period after each exercise. Use enough load to make the assigned repetitions challenging while maintaining good form. Unless otherwise specified, use the progression in table 9.30.

THE EXERCISES

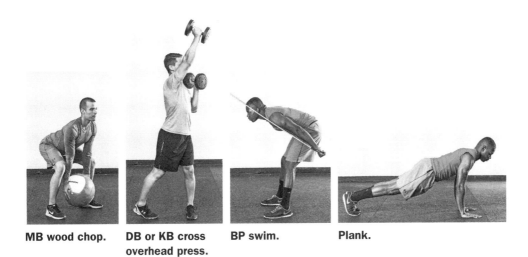

MB wood chop. DB or KB cross overhead press. BP swim. Plank.

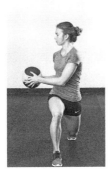

MB lunge with rotation.

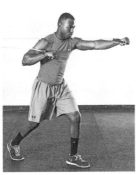

BP staggered-stance alternating press.

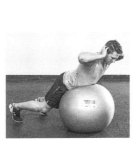

Recline pull (row).

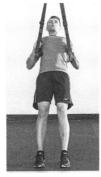

SB hyperextension.

> *continued*

THE HOW

If your fitness level is high, you can start with any week that feels comfortable and repeat the week as many times as necessary to create a strong base of training.

TABLE 9.30   Swimming: Conditioning Quadplexes

Exercise	Week 1	Week 2	Week 3	Week 4	Page
Quadplex 1 1. MB wood chop 2. DB or KB cross overhead press 3. BP swim 4. Plank	2 × 10	2 × 15	3 × 15	4 × 10 to 15	110 100 84 57
Quadplex 2 1. MB lunge with rotation 2. BP staggered-stance alternating press 3. Recline pull (row) 4. SB hyperextension	2 × 10	2 × 15	3 × 15	4 × 10 to 15	113 75 46 130

Core

Triple Threat (weeks 5-10): 1 or 2 sets

STRENGTH

Perform each quadplex in order for the number of sets indicated. Rest adequately between each exercise to maintain good form and quality of movement, eventually targeting a 30- to 60-second rest period after each exercise. Use enough load to make the assigned repetitions challenging while maintaining good form. Unless otherwise specified, use the progression in table 9.31.

Additional Warm-Up

Steel Core: 2 sets

THE EXERCISES

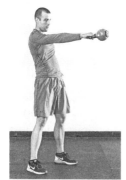
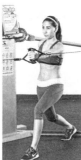
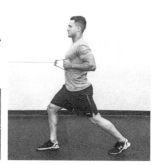
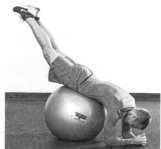

KB single-arm swing.   **BP push–pull.**   **BP staggered-stance CLA row.**   **SB reverse hyperextension.**

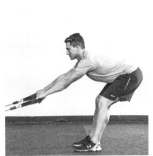
BP deadlift.

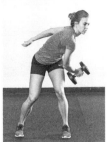
DB single-arm diagonal fly rotation.

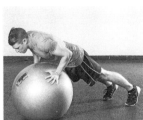
SB hands-on-ball push-up.

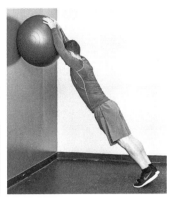
SB rollout.

THE HOW

If your fitness level is high, you can start with any week that feels comfortable and repeat the week as many times as necessary to create a strong base of training.

TABLE 9.31 Swimming: Strength Quadplexes

The KB single-arm swing and the DB single-arm diagonal fly rotation should be performed on each side.

Exercise	Week 1	Week 2	Week 3	Week 4	Page
Quadplex 1	1 × 6	2 × 6	3 × 4	4 × 4	
1. KB single-arm swing					91
2. BP push–pull					89
3. BP staggered-stance CLA row					81
4. SB reverse hyperextension					131
Quadplex 2	1 × 6	2 × 6	3 × 4	4 × 4	
1. BP deadlift					70
2. DB single-arm diagonal fly rotation					106
3. SB hands-on-ball push-up (slow)					125
4. SB rollout					127

Core

Triple Threat (weeks 11-15): 3 sets

POWER AND POWER ENDURANCE

Perform each biplex in order for the number of sets indicated. For power, rest 1 minute between the first and second exercises, and then rest 1 to 2 minutes between the second and first exercises. For power endurance, do not rest between the first and second exercises, and then rest 1 minute between the second and first exercises. Use enough load to make the assigned repetitions challenging while maintaining good form. Unless otherwise specified, use the progression in table 9.32.

Additional Warm-Up

Gary's Dumbbell Matrix: 2 sets

> continued

THE EXERCISES

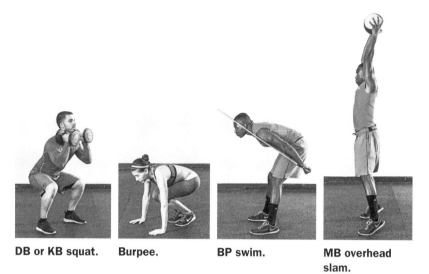

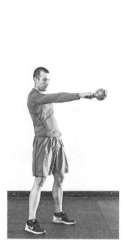

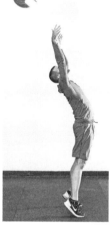

DB or KB squat.   **Burpee.**   **BP swim.**   **MB overhead slam.**

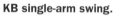

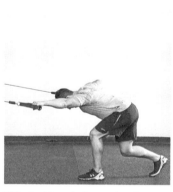

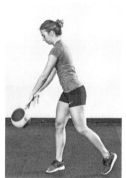

KB single-arm swing.   **MB reverse scoop throw.**   **BP staggered-stance bent-over alternating row.**   **MB overhead side-to-side slam.**

258

THE HOW

If your fitness level is high, you can start with any week that feels comfortable and repeat the week as many times as necessary to create a strong base of training.

TABLE 9.32 Swimming: Power and Power-Endurance Biplexes

The KB single-arm swing should be performed on each arm.

Exercise	Week 1	Week 2	Week 3	Week 4	Page
Biplex 1 1. DB or KB squat 2. Burpee	2 × 5 + 5	2 × 5 + 5	3 × 5 + 5	3 × 5 + 5	 90 68
Biplex 2 1. BP swim 2. MB overhead slam	2 × 5 + 5	2 × 5 + 5	3 × 5 + 5	3 × 5 + 5	 84 120
Biplex 3 1. KB single-arm swing 2. MB reverse scoop throw	2 × 5 + 5	2 × 5 + 5	3 × 5 + 5	3 × 5 + 5	 91 122

Biplex 4
1. BP staggered-stance bent-over
   alternating row
2. MB overhead side-to-side
   slam
	2 × 5 + 5	2 × 5 + 5	3 × 5 + 5	3 × 5 + 5	
					79
					
					121

5 + 5 indicates 60 seconds of rest between the first and second exercise for power. For power endurance, go straight from the first exercise to the second without resting.

Core

Triple Threat (weeks 15-20): 1 or 2 sets

SB hyperextension to SB reverse hyperextension: 2 × 10

Metabolic

If you need more cardio or metabolic training in the power-endurance phase, add interval cardio, such as 300-yard (274 m) shuttles (25 yd [22.8 m] × 12), to the end of the workout. Practice volume must be taken into account when prescribing more metabolic training.

Optional Metabolic Training

JC Meta Back: 2 or 3 sets

JC Leg Crank: 2 or 3 sets

Skating-related sports such as ice hockey and in-line skating require enormous rotational power from the hips and legs. Depending on the sport, the upper body can counterbalance the lower body during acceleration, maneuver a stick, or absorb impact. Regardless of how the upper body is used, the core is at the center of the coordination and synchronization between upper and lower body. It needs to provide rotational force transfer as well as stiffness for optimal force transfer.

Warm-Up for All Workouts

Chopper: 2 or 3 × 10

CONDITIONING

Perform each triplex in order and then start the sequence again. Complete as many sets as indicated. Rest adequately between each exercise to maintain good form and quality of movement, eventually targeting a 30- to 60-second rest period after each exercise. Use enough load to make the assigned repetitions challenging while maintaining good form. Unless otherwise specified, use the progression in table 9.33.

THE EXERCISES

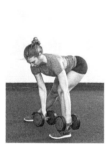

DB or KB lateral reaching lunge.

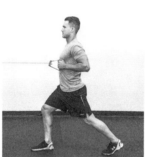

BP staggered-stance CLA row.

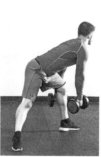

DB or KB upright row.

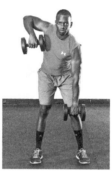

DB or KB rotating reaching lunge.

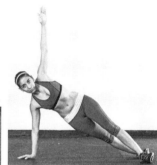

Side T plank.

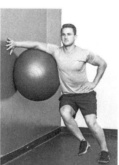

SB skier.

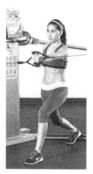

SB single-leg lateral wall slide.

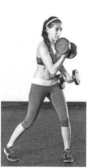

BP push–pull.

DB or KB cross uppercut.

THE HOW

If your fitness level is high, you can start with any week that feels comfortable and repeat the week as many times as necessary to create a strong base of training.

TABLE 9.33 Skating-Related Sports: Conditioning Triplexes

The SB single-leg lateral wall side should be performed on each leg.

Exercise	Week 1	Week 2	Week 3	Week 4	Page
Triplex 1	2 × 10	2 × 15	3 × 10 to 15	3 or 4 × 10 to 15	
1. DB or KB lateral reaching lunge					95
2. BP staggered-stance CLA row					81
3. DB or KB upright row (alternating)					103
Triplex 2	2 × 10	2 × 15	3 × 10 to 15	3 or 4 × 10 to 15	96
1. DB or KB rotating reaching lunge					
2. Side T plank (double-arm to single-arm progression)	10 to 30 sec.	10 to 30 sec.	10 to 30 sec.	10 to 30 sec.	58
3. SB skier	2 × 10	2 × 15	3 × 10 to 15	3 or 4 × 10 to 15	132
Triplex 3 (core)	2 × 10	2 × 15	3 × 10 to 15	3 or 4 × 10 to 15	
1. SB single-leg lateral wall slide					124
2. BP push–pull					89
3. DB or KB cross uppercut					104

Flush

Lateral slide: 2 or 3 × 10 to 20 reps per side

STRENGTH

Perform each triplex in order for the number of sets indicated. Rest adequately between each exercise to maintain good form and quality of movement, eventually targeting a 30- to 60-second rest period after each exercise. Use enough load to make the assigned repetitions challenging while maintaining good form. Unless otherwise specified, use the progression in table 9.34.

Additional Warm-Up

Gary's Dumbbell Matrix: 1 or 2 sets (1:2 work:rest ratio)

SB single-leg lateral wall slide: 2 or 3 × 10 per leg

> continued

THE EXERCISES

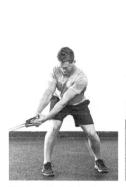

BP low-to-high chop.

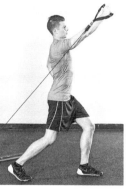

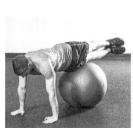

BP staggered-stance CLA incline press.

SB log roll.

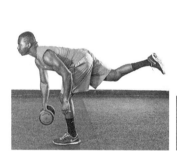

DB or KB single-leg RDL.

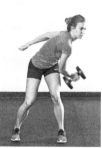

DB single-arm diagonal fly rotation.

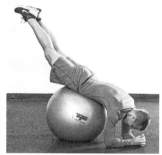

SB reverse hyperextension.

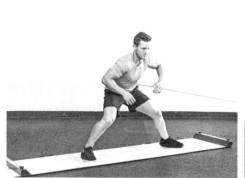

Lateral slide (band resistance).

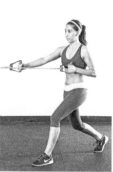

BP staggered-stance alternating row.

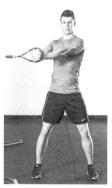

BP short rotation (10 to 2 o'clock).

THE HOW

If your fitness level is high, you can start with any week that feels comfortable and repeat the week as many times as necessary to create a strong base of training.

TABLE 9.34 Skating-Related Sports: Strength Triplexes

The DB or KB single-leg RDL and DB single-arm diagonal fly rotation should be performed on each side.

Exercise	Week 1	Week 2	Week 3	Week 4	Page
Triplex 1 1. BP low-to-high chop 2. BP staggered-stance CLA incline press 3. SB log roll	2 × 6	2 × 6	3 or 4 × 4	3 or 4 × 4	86 73 131
Triplex 2 1. DB or KB single-leg RDL 2. DB single-arm diagonal fly rotation 3. SB reverse hyperextension	2 × 6	2 × 6	3 or 4 × 4	3 or 4 × 4	92 106 131
Triplex 3 1. Lateral slide (band resistance) 2. BP staggered-stance alternating row 3. BP short rotation (10 to 2 o'clock)	2 × 6	2 × 6	3 or 4 × 4	3 or 4 × 4	140 78 87

Postworkout Flush

JC Leg Crank: 1 set

Skater: 2 or 3 sets of 10 to 20 reps per side

POWER AND POWER ENDURANCE

Perform each biplex in order for the number of sets indicated. For power, rest 1 minute between the first and second exercises, and then rest 1 to 2 minutes between the second and first exercises. For power endurance, do not rest between the first and second exercises, and then rest 1 minute between the second and first exercises. Use enough load to make the assigned repetitions challenging while maintaining good form. Unless otherwise specified, use the progression in table 9.35.

THE EXERCISES

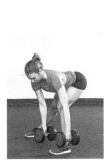
DB or KB lateral reaching lunge.

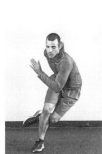
Skater.

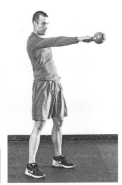
KB single-arm swing.

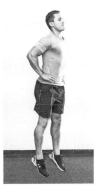
Squat jump.

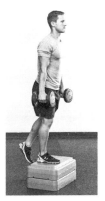
Loaded step-up.

> continued

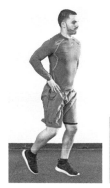

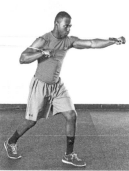

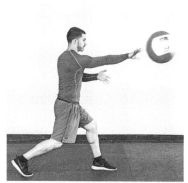

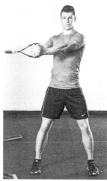

| Alternating split jump. | BP staggered-stance alternating press. | MB staggered-stance CLA straight chest throw. | BP short rotation (10 to 2 o'clock). |

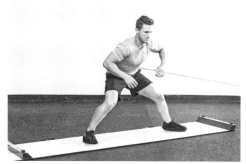

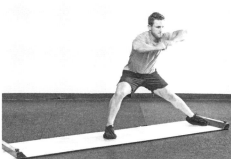

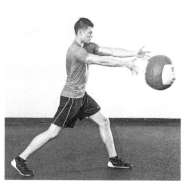

| Lateral slide (with band resistance). | Lateral slide. | MB rotational throw: perpendicular. |

THE HOW

If your fitness level is high, you can start with any week that feels comfortable and repeat the week as many times as necessary to create a strong base of training.

TABLE 9.35 Skating-Related Sports: Power and Power-Endurance Biplexes

The KB single-arm swing should be performed on each arm.

POWER					
Exercise	Week 1	Week 2	Week 3	Week 4	Page
Biplex 1 1. DB or KB lateral reaching lunge 2. Skater	2 × 5 + 5	2 × 5 + 5	3 × 5 + 5	3 × 5 + 5	95 67
Biplex 2 1. KB single-arm swing 2. Squat jump	2 × 5 + 5	2 × 5 + 5	3 × 5 + 5	3 × 5 + 5	91 66
Biplex 3 1. Loaded step-up (dumbbells) 2. Alternating split jump	2 × 5 + 5	2 × 5 + 5	3 × 5 + 5	3 × 5 + 5	55 66
Biplex 4 1. BP staggered-stance alternating press 2. MB staggered-stance CLA straight chest throw	2 × 5 + 5	2 × 5 + 5	3 × 5 + 5	3 × 5 + 5	75 118

Exercise	Week 1	Week 2	Week 3	Week 4	Page
Biplex 5	$2 \times 5 + 5$	$2 \times 5 + 5$	$3 \times 5 + 5$	$3 \times 5 + 5$	
1. BP short rotation (10 to 2 o'clock)					87
2. MB rotational throw: perpendicular					121
POWER ENDURANCE					
Biplex 1	$2 \times 5 + 10$	$2 \times 5 + 10$	$3 \times 5 + 10$	$3 \times 5 + 10$	
1. DB or KB lateral reaching lunge					95
2. Skater					67
Biplex 2	$2 \times 5 + 10$	$2 \times 5 + 10$	$3 \times 5 + 10$	$3 \times 5 + 10$	
1. KB single-arm swing					91
2. Squat jump					66
Biplex 3	$2 \times 5 + 10$	$2 \times 5 + 10$	$3 \times 5 + 10$	$3 \times 5 + 10$	
1. Loaded step up (dumbbells)					55
2. Alternating split jump					66
Biplex 4	$2 \times 5 + 10$	$2 \times 5 + 10$	$3 \times 5 + 10$	$3 \times 5 + 10$	
1. Lateral slide (with band resistance)					140
2. Lateral slide					140
Biplex 5	$2 \times 5 + 10$	$2 \times 5 + 10$	$3 \times 5 + 10$	$3 \times 5 + 10$	
1. BP short rotation (10 to 2 o'clock)					87
2. MB rotational throw: perpendicular					121

5 + 5 indicates 60 seconds of rest between the first and second exercise for power. For power endurance, go straight from the first exercise to the second without resting.

Postworkout Super Flush

Perform 2 or 3 sets with no rest:

JC Leg Crank

Lateral slide: 10 to 20 reps per side

Metabolic

If you need more cardio or metabolic training during the power-endurance phase, add interval cardio, such as 300-yard (274 m) shuttles (25 yd [22.8 m] × 12), to the end of the workout. Practice volume must be taken into account when prescribing more metabolic training.

Conclusion

The efficacy of functional training continues to be proven in gyms across the world while research from university laboratories attempts to explain the mechanisms behind its success. The functional training system in this book will allow the coach or athlete to improve athletic performance while minimizing the overuse problems often seen in traditional strength training—it offers the ability to train aggressively while not overloading and tearing down the body. In addition, the principle of specificity underlies the concept of functional training, providing the optimal training transfer to any sport.

Many other modalities and training philosophies have also stood the test of time. For this reason, the best approach to improve human performance is to take an eclectic view of training. The IHP Hybrid Training System is a systematic, comprehensive approach to combining the best practices in strength and conditioning in a simple, time-efficient manner.

I trust the information in this book has opened new doors to your performance-enhancement journey. It is my sincere wish that the work presented here will move the performance-enhancement industry forward, create stronger and healthier athletes, and lead to new avenues in future research.

Index

Note: The italicized *f* and *t* following page numbers refer to figures and tables, respectively.

About the Author

Juan Carlos Santana, MEd, CSCS, is the founder and director of the Institute of Human Performance (IHP) in Boca Raton, Florida. IHP has been recognized as one of the top training facilities in the world and the best core-training facility in the United States.

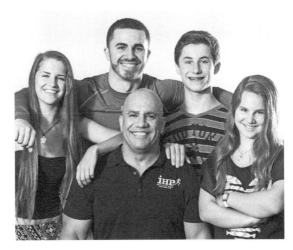

Santana has been part of the strength and conditioning programs for several Florida Atlantic University sports teams over the last two decades. He has been responsible for the strength and conditioning programs for men's basketball, men's and women's cross country, track and field, women's volleyball, and men's and women's swimming.

A member and certified strength and conditioning specialist with distinction (CSCS) and a Fellow (NSCAF) with the National Strength and Conditioning Association (NSCA). Santana is also a member and certified health fitness instructor with the ACSM. In addition, he is a certified senior coach and club coach course instructor with the U.S. weightlifting team and a level I coach with USA Track and Field.

Santana currently is on the NSCA Board of Directors and served 10 years as a sport-specific conditioning editor for the *NSCA Journal*. His professional responsibilities have included serving as NSCA vice president, chairman of the NSCA Coaches Conference, a member of the NSCA Conference Committee, and the NSCA Florida state director. As a college professor, he has taught strength and conditioning for the combat athlete, sports training systems, and strength training at Florida Atlantic University (FAU). He is an FAU graduate with bachelor's and master's degrees in exercise science and was the first graduate from FAU's exercise science department to receive the prestigious Alumni of the Year award in 2012. Santana is involved in several ongoing research studies with numerous universities.

Founded in 2001, IHP provides an unparalleled training environment for elite athletes, including Olympic athletes in a variety of sports; world-class tennis champions; NFL, NHL, and MLB players; world champion Brazilian jujitsu and mixed martial arts fighters; numerous NCAA Division I teams; and hundreds of nationally ranked teen hopefuls from a cross-section of sport disciplines.

To learn more about IHP's athlete training, products, and continuing education and functional training certificate programs for professionals, please visit www.ihpfit.com or www.ihpuniversity.com. For more information about functional training equipment, visit IHP partner Perform Better's website at www.performbetter.com.

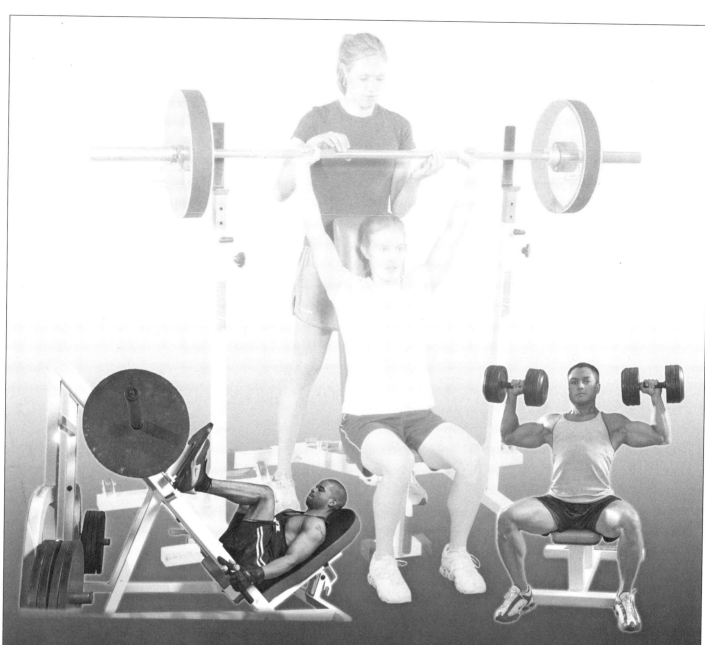

You'll find other outstanding strength training resources at

www.HumanKinetics.com/strengthtraining

In the U.S. call 1-800-747-4457

Australia 08 8372 0999 • Canada 1-800-465-7301
Europe +44 (0) 113 255 5665 • New Zealand 0800 222 062

HUMAN KINETICS
The Premier Publisher for Sports & Fitness
P.O. Box 5076 • Champaign, IL 61825-5076 USA